Palaeoepidemiology

Paleoseismology

Palaeoepidemiology

The Epidemiology of Human Remains

Tony Waldron

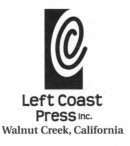

Left Coast Press Inc.
Walnut Creek, California

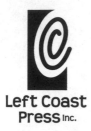

Left Coast
Press Inc.

Left Coast Press, Inc.
1630 North Main Street, #400
Walnut Creek, CA 94596
http://www.lcoastpress.com

ISBN 978-1-59874-252-7

Library of Congress Cataloging-in-Publication Data

Waldron, T. (Tony)
Paleoepidemiology : the measure of disease in the human past/Tony Waldron.
   p. ; cm.—(Publications of the Institute of Archaeology, University College London)
  Includes bibliographical references and index.
  ISBN-13: 978-1-59874-252-7 (hardback : alk. paper) 1. Paleopathology—Methodology.
2. Epidemiology. I. Title. II. Series.
[DNLM: 1. Paleopathology—methods. 2. Epidemiologic Methods. QZ 11.5 W167p 2007]
  R134.8.W353 2007   616.07072—dc22   2007025132

Printed in the United States of America

☉ The paper used in this publication meets the minimum requirements of American National Standard for Information Sciences—Permanence of Paper for Printed Library Materials, ANSI/NISO Z39.48–1992.

07 08 09 10 5 4 3 2 1

Left Coast Press Inc. is committed to preserving ancient forests and natural resources. We elected to print *Palaeoepidemiology* on 30% post consumer recycled paper, processed chlorine free. As a result, for this printing, we have saved:

   1 Trees (40' tall and 6-8" diameter)
   560 Gallons of Wastewater
  225 Kilowatt Hours of Electricity
   62 Pounds of Solid Waste
  121 Pounds of Greenhouse Gases

Left Coast Press Inc. made this paper choice because our printer, Thomson-Shore, Inc., is a member of Green Press Initiative, a nonprofit program dedicated to supporting authors, publishers, and suppliers in their efforts to reduce their use of fiber obtained from endangered forests.

For more information, visit www.greenpressinitiative.org

Contents

Preface

This book clarifies the application of epidemiological methods to the study of human remains, in particular, the study of disease in the past. I hope that it will encourage the proper use of epidemiology more widely in this field of study than has generally been the case.

The book is based on my earlier publication *Counting the Dead*,[1] and I am grateful to all those who read it and made comments for corrections and improvement. To no one am I more grateful than to Dr Neil Cheshire, who not only read it from cover to cover but also provided pages of corrigenda and suggestions, all of which I have incorporated here and which I have chosen not to acknowledge separately. Indeed, I would like to have had the courage, as did Austin Bradford Hill in the preface of the seventh edition (1961) of his *Principles of Medical Statistics*, to say of those who had proffered advice to him, sincerely to trust that the reader would hold them largely responsible for any faults that remained; but I can't quite do so. Instead I will admit that if there are good things about this book, they are largely due to the many discussions – formal and informal – I have had with friends and colleagues, and to my students who have corrected me when I have been more outrageous than normal during seminars and lectures. What errors there are, I own up to, but I hope for the opportunity to correct them in the future.

More than that, however, I hope that this book will be found to be informative and instructive and that parts of it may even be found to be entertaining.

Endnote

1. T. Waldron, *Counting the Dead* (Chichester: John Wiley & Sons, 1994).

Introduction

W hen I first became interested in the study of human remains, my day job was as an epidemiologist studying, among other things, the effects of toxic exposures in occupational groups, and so one of the main attractions of looking at skeletal assemblages was to see how the frequency of disease had fluctuated in the past. A number of problems quickly became apparent that did not seem to me to have been very greatly studied by others working in the area. As with so much of modern epidemiology, the problems were largely concerned with denominators, but there were others, including the nature of the material available for study and the difficulty in diagnosing disease in the skeleton.

The results of my deliberations over the years formed the basis of a small book published (I am astonished to find) over 10 years ago.[1] Since then I have continued to plague my colleagues and students, and, indeed, anyone else who will listen, with interminable exhortations to be more aware of the epidemiological implications of their work. I am extremely grateful that at least some of them continue to listen and that more of them than before now refer to prevalence, rather than incidence, when talking about the frequency of disease.

The book begins with a brief history of epidemiology, mostly modern, because there has been very little palaeoepidemiology until recently; most of those who study human remains having been content to work blissfully unaware of how it might help them. Most of the methods in common use in epidemiology have been developed in the last 40 or 50 years, and their development is briefly alluded to and some of the more significant figures in their history are given a mention. Palaeoepidemiological considerations are generally held to have started in a serious way with Hooton's study of the Pecos Indians, but a close examination of his methods shows that he was often seriously in error, as I attempt to demonstrate.

The difficulties encountered in palaeoepidemiology begin with the assemblages that are available for study, and these are considered in the second chapter. It is probably true to say that if modern epidemiologists had to work with the assemblages that bone specialists have at their disposal, they would quickly move on to another field of study, since almost nothing about them would satisfy their exacting requirements. If one insists on working with human remains, however, there is no hope that the archaeologists will provide anything more suitable, and so we must be content with what we have. The most serious imperfection in the assemblage is that almost everything about it is nonrandom, and its composition is almost completely beyond the control of the palaeoepidemiologists. Knowing this, however, may help to moderate the sometimes outrageous claims made for it, and this is the principal theme of this chapter.

Outcome variables are of the greatest importance in any epidemiological study; in palaeoepidemiology they are most often some disease or other condition that affects the skeleton and that requires diagnosis. It usually comes as a surprise to the nonmedical person that diagnosis is at best a very imprecise activity and is subject to fashions and vagaries to such an extent that repeated studies have shown that a substantial number of diagnoses – at least a quarter in some cases – is incorrect. It seems hardly likely that if modern clinicians, with all the aids at their disposal, are not very good diagnosticians, that those who examine human remains will be any better, given the limited amount of information that is available to them. This often disappoints the tyro, but some comfort can often be found from many of his or her colleagues, who have no doubts about their own ability to diagnose every condition in the skeleton, including some that are hardly recognised by modern medicine. In Chapter 3, I suggest that moderation rather than enthusiasm is a better approach to diagnosing disease in human remains and that in order to gain some consistency in the procedure it is better to produce operational definitions that can be commonly agreed on and universally used; despite several years of experience, I remain optimistic that this approach may eventually find general approval.

Chapters 4–7 are the heart of the matter and describe, firstly, methods that can be used to describe the frequency of disease in populations. In Chapter 4, I show that the only valid measure of frequency in palaeoepidemiology is prevalence and that the other measure commonly used in modern epidemiology – incidence – cannot be calculated, and neither can any other rate applied to modern populations, since they all include numbers of live individuals in the denominator. Difficulties in deciding appropriate denominators in palaeoepidemiology are discussed and approaches to overcome these difficulties suggested. This chapter also includes a note on the special problems associated with dental epidemiology.

Chapter 5 considers means of comparing prevalence among studies using either some form of standardisation or by calculating the common odds ratio. I come down in favour of using the common odds ratio for this purpose. In Chapter 6, I briefly discuss proportional morbidity and mortality, and ranking studies, which – since they do not use denominators – may sometimes overcome the difficulties in determining prevalence. The final chapter in this group, Chapter 7, introduces the reader to analytical methods in palaeoepidemiology, that is, when associations between different conditions are explored or when aetiological factors of disease are investigated. In this chapter the case-control study is described, and some examples of its use are given.

One feature of modern epidemiology is the trend toward increasingly complicating a subject that is, in fact, very simple and straightforward, usually through the use of mathematical symbols and equations that tend to frighten off those who thankfully left maths behind them as quickly as school examinations permitted. In this text statistics and mathematics have been kept to a minimum, and even the most extreme 'arithmophobe'[2] should find nothing to produce panic or anxiety. My intention here is to point out the major pathways through rather troublesome terrain; those who wish for more detailed information on the topography will need larger scale maps. They will do well to consult some of the epidemiological texts referred to here.

Chapter 8 deals with the suggestion that it is possible to deduce occupation from the skeleton. This seemed a very attractive proposition when I initially started to examine human remains, but it quickly became apparent that the notion was fatally flawed. The idea has roots in the many epidemiological studies of – for example – the development of osteoarthritis in different occupations, but it is clear that some of those who support it have ignored the negative evidence or lack the necessary epidemiological experience to spot the weakness in their case. In this chapter I show that occupation can*not* be deduced from lesions in the skeleton, a fact that my students are usually able to grasp in very short order. I do not expect that those who wish it otherwise will be persuaded by my arguments, but I do hope to put doubts in the minds of those who are not committed to the notion, so that they will view claims that are made about the activities of our ancestors with a good deal of scepticism. In this context we should remember, with Francis Bacon, that 'what a man would like to be true, he more readily believes'.[3]

The final chapter brings together the various strands in other chapters to suggest the essentials in planning an epidemiological study based on human remains. Attention is given to preparing protocols and procedures well in advance of beginning the study; to producing operational definitions of outcome variables; to the importance of inter- and intraobserver tests; to ways to avoid bias as far as possible; and the need to keep the analysis of results as simple as possible. I also make the radical suggestion that a statistician should be involved in planning the study at the outset and that it is often no bad thing to get some advice from an epidemiologist if there are any doubts about the collective skills within the study group.

Endnotes

1. T. Waldron, *Counting the Dead* (Chichester: John Wiley & Sons, 1994).

2. I am grateful for this term to Dr Neil Cheshire. who kindly corrected an earlier effort!

3. *Quod enim mavult homo verum esse, id potius credit, Novum Organum*, Book I, Aphorism 49.

1 | The Development of Epidemiology

Curiosity about the nature and the cause of disease has been apparent throughout human history, and there is no reason to suppose that the same was not true for those of our ancestors for whom we have no written records. The earliest explanations for illness were couched in magical or religious terms, and it was to the priest or shaman that the sick looked for cures either by propitiating the gods or demons who had induced the illness,[1] or by countering spells that had been placed on the sick individual.[2] The most influential theory of disease was proposed some time in the fourth century BCE and attributed to the school of Hippocrates of Cos (*ca* 460–377 BCE). This was the doctrine of the humours, which held that the state of health – eucrasia – depended on the correct balance of the four humours in the body: blood, phlegm, bile, and black bile. Illness – or dyscrasia – supervened when the balance was disturbed, by dietary or environmental factors,[3] for example, and the role of the physician was to restore the balance either by restoring the humours that were lacking or by removing those that were in excess; these objectives would be achieved by means of dietary adjustments or medicines, or by blood letting or purging. The belief in this doctrine was reinforced by the teachings of Galen (*ca* 130–200), a Greek physician who practiced in Rome in the second century CE, which held sway well into the early modern period and lingered well beyond; remnants are to be found to this day. We may still describe an individual as being phlegmatic, and many of our mothers and grandmothers were heard to say that they had a bilious headache; the modern day haematologist may also decide that a patient has a blood dyscrasia or a bleeding diathesis.

The roots of what we can recognise as truly modern medicine are embedded in eighteenth-century soil, particularly in the rise of anatomy and of the autopsy. During the late eighteenth and early nineteenth centuries physicians followed their patients to the mortuary to try to find the alterations in the normal anatomy of the organs of the body that might explain their symptoms. When physical examination was augmented by tools such as the stethoscope, the sounds heard in the chest during life were assessed in the light of changes found in the heart and lungs at autopsy. First in Paris and then in Vienna, the great schools of pathological anatomy flourished during the nineteenth century.[4] The microscope ushered in further developments in medical thought; Rudolf Virchow (1821–1902) proposed the cellular theory of pathology, and his younger contemporary Robert Koch (1843–1910) did much to propagate the bacterial aetiology of disease, most particularly through the discovery of the tubercle bacillus and the adumbration of his postulates.[5] In more recent times we have discovered viruses, abnormal immune responses, and imperfect genes on which to blame our ailments, but we are still little better than the Greeks at preventing them.

The notion that clues to the cause of disease might come from observing who got what, when, and where – in other words, from the study of the epidemiology of disease – was a Johnny-come-lately to the medical party. The first serious attempt to examine patterns in recorded mortality was made by John Graunt, a haberdasher in London, who examined trends in the London *Bills of Mortality*.[6] The *Bills* were first published in 1592 following an outbreak of plague but rapidly fell into disuse, being revived again in 1603, another plague year. They were published weekly, on a Thursday, and on the Thursday before Christmas a yearly compilation was published, a timely reminder of the manifest conditions to which Londoners would one day succumb – and probably sooner rather than later.[7] In each of the London parishes, when a death was announced by the tolling of a bell, or by informing the sexton, the sexton informed the searchers ('antient Matrons sworn to their office'),[8] who would visit the corpse and determine as best they could the cause of death, being somewhat hampered in their task by a lack of medical training. The searchers then informed the parish clerk of their conclusions, and each Tuesday he, in turn, informed the clerk of the Hall of the happenings during the preceding week; the various accounts were compiled on Wednesday, published on Thursday, and delivered to all those who chose to pay four shillings a year for them.

When Graunt analysed the causes of death, he noted, for example, that in almost all the years between 1629 and 1660, consumption accounted for at least one fifth of all deaths.[9] He contrasted the number of deaths and christenings among parishes and between sexes and, like a good epidemiologist, was generally aware of the potential errors and biases in his data.

The publication of Graunt's book in 1664 was followed by many decades of silence, the next important developments being stimulated by the provision of data from the decennial censuses that began in 1801 and the compulsory registration of births, deaths, and marriages, starting in 1837 – and by the great cholera epidemics. There were four cholera epidemics during the nineteenth century: 1831–2, 1848–9, 1853–4, and 1865–6, each resulting in considerable mortality.[10] It was during the third epidemic in 1854 that John Snow (1813–1858) famously removed the handle from the Broad Street pump in London to demonstrate that the disease was waterborne;[11] this action is often seen as the gestational act that signalled the birth of epidemiology, although the London Epidemiological Society[12] had been founded a few years earlier (in 1850), initially to direct anti-cholera activities, and there were others who had been carrying out work, on earlier epidemics, that would nowadays be described as epidemiological in nature.[13]

Snow's status among modern epidemiology has reached almost mythic proportions,[14] and although it is true that he demonstrated cholera to be a waterborne disease, his theory was not widely held in his own time. He was rather better known in his own time as an anaesthetist, administering chloroform to Queen Victoria during the birth of her eighth and ninth children, Prince Leopold in 1853 and Princess Beatrice in 1857.[15]

Although Snow is generally credited as being the father of epidemiology, a better claim for paternity in my view can be made for William Farr (1808–1883), who was Collator of Abstracts at the office of the Registrar General from 1838–1878, having been passed over for the post of Registrar General the preceding year.[16] Farr analysed the data collected by the Registrar General and published summary accounts from time to time, including decennial occupational mortality tables from 1861 onward, which invariably showed the baneful effect of work on the expectation of life. Farr was not always very sympathetic toward those whose deaths were accelerated by their occupation – stating, for example, that if publicans wished to live as long as others 'they have only to abstain from excesses in spirits and other strong drinks', exemplifying the British characteristic of disapproving of those provide them with their pleasures.

Edwin Chadwick (1800–1890) had previously found that the average age at which labourers might die in Manchester might be as low as 17, whereas that of the gentry in Rutlandshire was 52.[17] Chadwick's thesis was that the explanation for the difference lay in the insanitary physical conditions in which the labouring poor lived; he ignored the effects of occupation and thus perpetuated a schism between public and occupational health that has persisted to the present day.[18] There were other attempts to study the effects of work on health during the nineteenth century, when working conditions were as bad as they have ever been, including those of Daniel Noble, a supporter of the factory system to which, he concluded from his own studies, that 'no peculiar evils [necessarily] attach'.[19]

The most important epidemiological methods, including prospective and case-control studies, were developed and refined in the middle years of the last century,[20] and these went hand in hand with new statistical methods that were increasingly applied to epidemiological analysis.[21] Methods of dealing with complicating factors, such as confounding, were also elaborated in the second half of the twentieth century.[22] The trend has generally been to take what are basically simple techniques and concepts and make them more complicated with the aid of seemingly complex algebra and jargon.

Once of the most interesting statisticians in the history of epidemiology was Austin (Tony) Bradford Hill, who contributed in a fundamental way to dealing with the problem of causality;[23] that is, when can one be reasonably certain that an effect that is observed with exposure to a particular substance is a causal relationship rather than a mere association? This is a problem that arises especially in occupational epidemiology: large populations exposed to potentially toxic substances provide epidemiologists with ideal material to study.[24]

In 1965 Bradford Hill published, in the relatively obscure *Journal of the Royal Society of Medicine*, what has become one of the most frequently cited papers in epidemiology. (It was, in fact, his inaugural address as president of the Society's section of occupational medicine.) In this paper[25] Bradford Hill listed nine features that he believed should be taken into account when trying to answer the question posed in the title of his talk,[26] which is one of the central problems in epidemiology, old or new. Since their publication, these nine 'features to be considered'[27] have become widely known and used as Bradford Hill's criteria. Bradford Hill would have been astounded had he known this would be the consequence of his efforts, since he expressed the views that none would provide indisputable evidence for or against a cause-and-effect relationship and that cause and effect could not even be decided by a set of rules.[28] The emphasis on these 'criteria' and their misapplication[29] has led to some other important aspects in the paper being ignored;[30] the paper remains required reading for any epidemiologist, however, whether dealing with modern or ancient populations.

The Epidemiology of Human Remains

Modern epidemiology pays not the slightest attention to human remains, and what little attention has been given to them has been as an adjunct to palaeopathology. The earliest palaeopathological studies were largely descriptive, detailing findings in interesting individual cases or groups of cases, mostly according to the medical model; this practice has continued to the present day and provides a substantial proportion of all publications in the field. An important new phase in palaeopathology was signalled by the publication of Earnest Hooton's study of the Pecos Indians in 1930.[31] Roney, writing in 1959,[32] saw Hooton's study as ushering in what he called the fourth stage of palaeopathology, that of the palaeoepidemiological study.[33] The importance of Hooton's work was not in the results that he obtained – which were not very informative, as we shall see – but in his attempt to apply population statistics to the material he studied.

Despite the ringing endorsements, Hooton actually devoted very little space either to palaeopathology (25 of the 391 pages) or to what can be called the epidemiological aspects (all summarised in 10 tables). The great bulk of the work was taken up with aspects of the skull, its measurements, morphology, and morphological types; probably not surprising since anthropologists were still in the grip of what Jarcho has referred to as a cranial fixation, which has by no means disappeared.[34]

Hooton[35] described few pathological conditions but did include one that he called spondylitis deformans, which ranged from marginal osteophytosis to extensive ankylosis; it is clear that this is not a single aetiological entity but presumably included conditions such as ankylosing spondylitis and diffuse idiopathic skeletal hyperostosis (DISH) among others. In Table X-I, on page 307, he presented data that at first glance seem to be the prevalence of spondylitis deformans by age (Table 1.1). As can be seen from Table 1.1, however, he is actually presenting two different things: first, the number of cases in each

Table 1.1 Reported prevalence of spondylitis deformans in Pecos Indians, by age[a]

In row 1, the prevalence is calculated using the total number of those with spondylitis deformans (132) as the denominator. In row 2, the denominator is the total number in the population (503)

		Age	
	Young Adult (21–35 years)	Middle-Aged (36–50 years)	Old (> 50 years)
1 Percent of total affected	3.03	34.85	62.12
2 Percent of total population	0.40	4.57	8.15

[a]Data abstracted from Hooton (1930).

age group as a proportion of the total population (n = 503), which seems to include subadults as well as adults; second, the number of cases by age as a proportion of the total number of cases. In other tables in his book (for example, X-2, which shows similar data for osteoarthritis in extraspinal sites), Hooton concludes that the incidence is greater in some groups than in others. As Chapter 3 in this book indicates, Hooton is in error in referring to the incidence of a condition in this context, since prevalence is the correct term (although to do him justice, he uses both terms indiscriminately), but he is not recording prevalence since he is using the wrong denominator (the total number in the population, or the total number of cases).

In Table 1.1 there appears to be a doubling of the frequency in the old, compared with the middle-aged group. If the prevalence is actually calculated – and this is not quite as easy as it might be since Hooton does not provide the data required, which have to be estimated from those he does – then the approximate results, together with the 95% confidence intervals (CI), are shown in Table 1.2.[36] The prevalence in the young and middle-aged groups is not significantly

Table 1.2 Prevalence (% and 95% confidence intervals) of spondylitis deformans in Pecos Indians, by age[a]

	Age Group		
	Young Adult	Middle-Aged	Old
Prevalence (%)	2.4	9.6	33.3
95% confidence interval	0.7–8.5	6.5–14.0	25.6–42.1

[a]Data abstracted from Hooton (1930). Age groups as shown in Table 1.1. See text for determination of denominators.

different (since the 95% CI overlap), but the prevalence in the old-age group is now almost three and a half times that of the middle-age group, and this is a statistically significant difference.

Roney pointed to a number of studies other than Hooton's that had used population statistics to estimate the prevalence of disease or to calculate expectations of life,[37] and he made a contribution himself through his account of the pathology found in the human remains excavated from a site in California, calculating prevalence rates for a number of conditions.[38]

Although Hooton's paper did not usher in the start of a fruitful period of palaeoepidemiology, there was an epidemiological thread in much of the work that was carried out in the 1960s and 1970s, although what might be called the interpretative influence was greatest. This influence has tended to become increasingly the trend as the medical input into the subject has been diluted; the performance of some exponents of interpretative palaeopathology is such as to suggest, in Isaiah Berlin's wonderful phrase, that 'their gifts lay in other spheres'.[39]

The urge to provide a good story for one's readers is so tempting as to be well nigh impossible to resist by many who study human remains, and, although this may make for better reading than a more factual report, it also makes for less rigorous work, is less intellectually challenging, and does not do enough to take the discipline beyond the realm of myth and fable.

One of the most interesting aspects of palaeopathology is the process of determining the way in which the frequency of disease has changed over time and in different parts of the world. Through this process we may learn something about the aetiology of disease, but such knowledge can be achieved only through the use of appropriate epidemiological tools. I hope that those who read this book will find themselves well on their way to reaching this goal.

Endnotes

1. If the interpretation of figures in some palaeolithic paintings as magicians or sorcerers is correct, the shaman was evidently a significant figure in prehistoric society in Europe; it was presumably to shamans that early man turned when ill. [See J. Clottes and N. Lewis-Williams, *Les chamanes de la préhistoires. Transe et magie dans les grottes ornées* (Paris: Seuil, 1996)].

2. For further details see H. Sigerist, *A History of Medicine, Volume I: Primitive and Archaic Medicine* (New York: Oxford University Press, 1951) (especially pp. 125–141).

3. The Hippocratic school was the first – or at least the first for which we have written evidence – to link health with the environment. [See Hippocrates, *Airs, Waters, Places,*

trans. W. H. S. Jones (Cambridge, MA: Harvard University Press, Loeb Classical Library, 1923)].

4. In Vienna the lucky patient was said to be the one who was cared for in hospital during life by Josef Skoda (1805–1881) and then studied in death by Karl Rokitanski (1804–1878); how one described the patient who managed to escape cured from hospital is not clear.

5. Koch's postulates lay down the criteria necessary to establish that an infectious agent causes a particular disease: The organism must be present in all infected individuals; it must be isolated from them and grown in culture; a pure culture must cause the disease in susceptible animals and be removed from them and regrown in culture. The postulates are still used to determine the aetiology of disease, in the discussion of HIV as the causative agent of AIDS, for example [V. Harden, 'Koch's Postulates and the Etiology of AIDS: An Historical Perspective', *History and Philosophy of the Life Sciences* 14 (1992): 249–69)]. Further details of Koch's life and work can be found in R. Munch, 'Robert Koch', *Microbes and Infection* 5 (2003): 69–74.

6. Graunt was born in London in 1620 and was elected to the Fellowship of the Royal Society in 1663. He died in 1674 and was buried at St Dunstan's in Fleet Street under the pews on the north side of the middle aisle. There has been no biography of Graunt, but a short account of his life was published by John Aubrey, who noted 'what pitty 'tis so great an ornament of the city should be buryed so obscurely!' [*Brief Lives and Other Selected Writings*, ed. Anthony Powell (New York: Charles Scribner's Sons, 1949), pp. 275–6].

7. Causes of death were first included in the *Bills* in 1624, together with a breakdown of the number of deaths according to sex.

8. John Graunt, *Natural and Political Observations Mentioned in a following Index, and made upon the Bills of Mortality* (London: Thomas Rycroft and Thomas Dicas, 1662), p. 13.

9. Those who died of consumption were sometimes reported by the searchers to be 'very lean and worn away' (Graunt, p. 14). Some of these individuals may have died from other wasting diseases such as diabetes, thyrotoxicosis, and malignant disease, but the great majority would almost certainly have died of tuberculosis.

10. The number of deaths in each of the epidemics has been estimated (in round figures) as 31,000, 58,000, 19,000, and 14,000 for the first to fourth, respectively. [C. H. Collins, 'Cholera Epidemics in 19th-Century Britain', *The Biomedical Scientist* 48 (2004): 141–43].

11. Snow removed the pump handle when the epidemic was waning, so the action seems to have had little or no effect on the disease [K. S. McLeod, 'Our Sense of Snow: The Myth of John Snow in Medical Geography', *Social Science and Medicine* 50 (2000): 923–35].

12. The term *epidemiologist*, however, does not seem to have been used until the 1860s, those people carrying out epidemiological work still, presumably, clinging to the notion that such work was part of their normal activities as physicians.

13. G. Davey Smith and S. Ebrahim, 'Epidemiology – Is It Time to Call It a Say? *International Journal of Epidemiology* 1 (2001): 1–11.

14. There are – interestingly – relatively few biographies of him: the best is P. Vinter-Johnson, H. Brody, N. Paneth, S. Rachman, and M. Rip, *Cholera, Chloroform, and the Science of Medicine* (Oxford: Oxford University Press, 2003).

15. *The Lancet* was substantially unimpressed by what it called the 'rumour' that Queen Victoria had chloroform during labour. It deplored the 'unnecessary inhalation', fearing that the Royal example might be followed 'with extraordinary readiness by a certain class of society'; no prizes for guessing the sex of the author of this piece (Editorial, *The Lancet*, 1853, i, 453).

16. In this office, Farr was, in effect, the nation's chief vital statistician. He was born in Shropshire in 1807 and qualified as an apothecary in 1832. He set up practice in Grafton Street in London and became friendly with Sir James Clark, a distinguished physician, and Thomas Wakley, the founder of the *Lancet*; it was through their good offices that he probably secured his post in the Registrar's Office. He died in 1883, having been elected to the Fellowship of the Royal Society in 1855 and awarded an honorary MD by the University of Oxford two years later. [See J. M. Eyler, *Victorian Social Medicine: The Ideas and Methods of William Farr* (Baltimore, MD: Johns Hopkins University Press, 1979)]. His thesis on the causation of cholera – that it was inversely related to the mean elevation above the high-water mark in London – was much more acceptable to his contemporaries than Snow's [J. M. Eyler, 'The Changing Assessment of John Snow's and William Farr's Cholera Studies', *Sozial- und Präventivmedizin* 46 (2001): 225–32].

17. Chadwick's data have generally been ignored by historians and statisticians alike; an attempt to rehabilitate them is given by J. Hanley, 'Edwin Chadwick and the Poverty of Statistics', *Medical History* 46 (2002): 21–40.

18. Chadwick is best known for his work as Secretary for the Poor Law Commission, to which post he was appointed in 1832. In 1842 he published privately his *Report into the Sanitary Conditions among the Working Classes,* in which he proposed *inter alia* the separation of drinking water from sewage. He was a difficult character and not much liked; '... he must have been an aggravating colleague, and the inevitable cause of much friction and irritation', wrote *The Times* on his death (7 July 1890). The writer did concede, however, that 'few men [had done] better work in his own special departments', but his irascibility was almost certainly the reason that his knighthood was delayed to the year before his death.

19. D. Noble, *Facts and Observations Relative to the Influence of Manufactures on Health and Life* (London: John Churchill, 1843), p. 78. Noble carried out one of the first occupational epidemiological studies, examining 50 children who worked in factories and 50 who worked in other occupations or not at all. Eight of the factory children were in 'bad' health compared with three of the others. Although the proportion of factory children in bad health is almost three times greater than in the other children (16% compared with 6%, respectively), it is a nonsignificant result. It is interesting that Noble carried out the study blind as to the status of the children, 'anxious to avoid entertaining any bias with respect to the issue' (Noble, p. 54), but he was also blind to the other flaws in his study.

20. E. Susser and M. Bresnahan, 'Origins of Epidemiology', *Annals of the New York Academy of Sciences* 954 (2001): 6–18; R. Doll, 'Cohort Studies: History of the Method. I. Prospective Cohort Studies', *Sozial- und Präventivmedizin* 46 (2001): 75–86; 'II. Retrospective Cohort Studies', *Ibid.,* 152–60; N. Paneth, E. Susser, and M. Susser, 'Origins and Development of the Case-Control Study: Part 1, Early Evolution', *Sozial- und Präventivmedizin* 47 (2002): 282–88; 'Part 2, the Case-Control Study from Lane-Claypon to 1950', *Ibid.,* 359–65.

21. A. Hardy and M. E. Magnello, 'Statistical Methods in Epidemiology: Karl Pearson, Ronald Ross, Major Greenwood, and Austin Bradford Hill, 1900–1945', *Sozial- und Präventivmedizin* 47 (2002): 80–89.

22. J. P. Vandenbroucke, 'The History of Confounding', *Sozial- und Präventivmedizin* 47 (2002): 216–24.

23. Bradford Hill (1897–1991) was the son of a famous father, Sir Leonard Hill, professor of physiology at the London Hospital. He had intended to follow a medical career but contracted tuberculosis during the First World War and read economics and then statistics instead. He worked at the statistical division of the Medical Research Council's National Institute of Medical Research before joining the staff of the London School of Hygiene and Tropical Medicine in 1927, eventually becoming professor of medical statistics in 1945, a post he retained until his retirement in 1961. He is famous among medical statisticians for having devised the randomized clinical trial (RCT) to test the efficacy of streptomycin in the treatment of tuberculosis ['Streptomycin Treatment of Tuberculosis, *British Medical Journal* 2 (1948): 769–83]; the RCT remains the definitive method of drug testing to the present day [P. Armitage, 'Obituary: Sir Austin Bradford Hill', *Journal of the Royal Statistical Society, Series A* 154 (1991): 482–84]. He collaborated with Richard Doll (1912–2005) in examining the relationship between smoking and lung cancer. These results were presented in a series of papers, the most famous being that which first reported on a large prospective study [R. Doll and A. Bradford Hill, 'The Mortality of Doctors in Relation to Their Smoking Habits. A Preliminary Study', *British Medical Journal* 2 (1950): 739–48]. It was this study that set Doll off on a career that ended in his becoming the best-known medical epidemiologist in the world [C. Richmond, 'Sir Richard Doll', *British Medical Journal* 331 (2005): 295]. In 1937 Bradford Hill published what is still the only textbook on medical statistics that can be read for pleasure and that went through 11 editions in his lifetime [*Principles of Medical Statistics* (London: The Lancet)].

24. S. D. Stellman, 'Issues of Causality in the History of Occupational Epidemiology', *Sozial- und Präventivmedizin* 48 (2003): 151–60.

25. A. Bradford Hill, 'The Environment and Disease: Association or Causation?' *Journal of the Royal Society of Medicine* 58 (1965): 295–300.

26. These were strength of the association; consistency; specificity; temporality; toxicological gradient; plausibility; coherence; experiment; and analogy.

27. A. Bradford Hill, p. 296.

28. Rothman and Greenland go so far as to suggest that there are *no* causal criteria at all in epidemiology [K. Rothman and S. Greenland, 'Causation and Causal Inference in Epidemiology', *American Journal of Public Health* 95 (2005): S144–50].

29. M. Höfler, 'The Bradford Hill Consideration on Causality: A Counterfactual Perspective', *Emerging Themes in Epidemiology* 2 (2005): 11–19.

30. C. V. Phillips and K. J. Goodman, 'The Missed Lesson of Sir Austin Bradford Hill', *Epidemiological Perspectives and Innovations* 1 (2004): 3–7.

31. E. A. Hooton, *The Indians of Pecos Pueblo. A Study of Their Skeletal Remains* (New Haven, CT: Yale University Press, 1930).

32. J. G. Roney, 'Palaeopathology of a Californian Archaeological Site', *Bulletin of the History of Medicine* 33 (1959): 97–109.

33. The first three stages had been outlined by Léon Pales (1905–1988). The first, from 1774 to 1870, was given to the study of quarternary animals; the second, from 1870 to 1900, was concerned with traumatic lesions and research into the origins of syphilis; the third, post-1900 stage was characterised by research into other infectious diseases [L. Pales, *Palèopathologie et pathologie comparative* (Paris: Masson, 1930)]. Laurence

Angel (1915–1986), in his history of palaeopathology, differs from Pales somewhat: he included everything up to the turn of the twentieth century as a first phase, ushering in a second, creative phase that ended with the First World War. In Angel's scheme there followed a period of depression that was reversed by Hooton [J. L. Angel, 'History and Development of Paleopathology', *American Journal of Physical Anthropology* 56 (1981): 509–15].

34. S. Jarcho, 'The Development and Present Condition of Palaeopathology in the United States', in *Human Palaeopathology*, ed. S. Jarcho (New Haven, CT: Yale University Press, 1966), pp. 3–30.

35. Earnest Hooton (1887–1954), that 'witty and genial man' (Jarcho, p. 22), was best known for his anthropometric work. His interest in the skeleton seems to have developed when he was a Rhodes Scholar in Oxford, and then working for a while with Arthur Keith in the Hunterian Museum of the Royal College of Surgeons of London. On his return to the United States he was offered a post at Harvard, where he remained, in the Peabody Museum, for the next 40 years. He excelled as a teacher and as a supervisor of graduate students. He was a founding member of the American Association of Physical Anthropology and associate editor of the *American Journal of Physical Anthropology* from 1928–1942 [S. M. Garn and E. Gils, 'Earnest Albert Hooton', *Biographical Memoirs* 68 (1996): 167–79].

36. Hooton based his results in Table X-1 on a total group of 503 individuals, although he reports earlier in the book (p. 18) that 594 individuals were actually aged. He does not say how the 503 were chosen from the base population, but in calculating the prevalence I have assumed that the distribution of ages in the smaller group is the same as in the larger. The prevalence so calculated is, thus, only approximate, but it ought not to be too far from the 'true' prevalence, assuming there was no bias in selecting the group for the palaeopathological study.

37. Among those whom Roney picked out for special mention were Krogman, Angel, Goldstein, Vallois, and Todd; the references to the specific papers are to be found in Roney's 1959 paper, pp. 108–09.

38. Roney's main conclusions are found in his 1959 paper, but they were also published in an abbreviated form in 1966, with an interesting discussion by A. M. Bunes, S. F. Cook, and J. E. Anderson [J. G. Roney, 'Palaeoepidemiology: An example from California', in *Human Palaeopathology*, ed. S. Jarcho (New Haven, CT: Yale University Press, 1966), pp. 99–107, discussion pp. 107–29].

39. I. Berlin, *Personal Impressions*, ed. H. Hardy (Oxford: Oxford University Press, 1982), p. 146.

Everyone presumably agrees that a collection of human remains is an assemblage, but what else it might represent is less clear. Is it a population; is it a sample? If neither, what is it? The epidemiological nature of the assemblage will now be discussed.

Populations

Modern epidemiology concerns itself with the study of disease in the living; the unit of study is a population that, for example, might be all the women in South Wales, workers in a factory, children in primary schools in Manchester. Almost any group runs the risk of attracting the attentions of the epidemiologist. The characteristic of all these populations, however, is that they are composed entirely of living individuals,[1] and it is axiomatic in epidemiology that the study populations are alive, although they also have other characteristics: in particular, they may be closed or open.

Closed Populations

A closed population is one in which there is no flow of individuals into or out of it. This situation has the inevitable consequence that the population will diminish in number over time and eventually die out. A closed population rarely occurs outside the mind of an epidemiologist or a demographer, but it does form the basis for the calculation of life tables.

Open Populations

By contrast, an open population permits loss and gain in number through the agency of births, deaths, immigration, and emigration. This situation is readily recognised as the more normal state of affairs. An open population may be *stable* if loss and gain are balanced so that the net effect is a relatively constant population size; in a *dynamic* population, in contrast, imbalance in gain and loss is the norm, so the population size varies over time. Dynamic, open populations are those most usually encountered in real life and in normal epidemiological practice.

Samples. Observations of a disease's behaviour in a community are sometimes made, and an intervention of some kind might be instigated – for example, limiting exposure to a potentially toxic agent, introducing a new treatment, or introducing (or abandoning) a vaccination programme. It is usually not practicable to study an entire population, and so a smaller group – a sample – is usually selected; the results from the sample are then extrapolated to the wider population from which the sample was drawn. A major part in the planning of any modern epidemiological investigation is taken up with ensuring that, in order to avoid bias, the sample being studied is representative of the larger group from which it is taken. In this way, one hopes that the results will be valid and that any actions taken on the basis of the study will be truly justified and produce the desired beneficial effect. Bias, that is, systematic error, is the bane of modern epidemiology; errors are inevitable and acceptable since one can usually rely on the statisticians to provide the necessary corrective measures; but bias, which disturbs the outcome of the study, is difficult to control, often unpredictable, and can be hard to detect.[2]

Paleoepidemiologists are fortunate in so far as they do not need to suffer from any anxieties that their work may have unfortunate, perhaps even dangerous, consequences for those they study, since the worst they can do is to cause some misleading information to appear in the journals that accept their work; they are not likely adversely to affect public health policy, or alter prescribing habits, or lead to the banning of potentially dangerous work practices. However, they do owe it to themselves and their potential editors and readers to consider sources of bias in their work and to plan and interpret their investigations with biases in mind.[3]

In modern practice, samples for epidemiological study are typically drawn at random.[4] The methods employed in drawing a random sample vary, but they should ensure that – in theory, at least – each member of the population has an equal chance of being selected. In practice, true random selection can be extremely difficult; even the generation of a list of random numbers with the aid of a computer is not without its problems.[5] What tends to happen in practice is that some quasi-random procedure is adopted – for example, selecting individuals from a nominal roll such as a telephone book, or a trade or profession directory, using a set of random numbers. Sources of bias in such a strategy are clear, the most obvious being that those excluded from such rolls have no chance of being selected and those who *are* included may – and sometimes *will* – differ in many respects from those who are not.[6] One reason for using less than perfect sampling methods, including using volunteers,[7] is that there are usually constraints on any epidemiological study, the principal ones being the time allotted to the study and the amount of money available to fund it. Nevertheless, if the sample is selected properly and with care, the chances of one source of bias – selection bias – should be greatly reduced, although probably not entirely eliminated, and the results will be that much more reliable.

It should be clear that an assemblage of human remains is neither a population nor a sample,[8] since it is neither living nor a random selection of those who were once living; indeed, almost everything about it is *non*random, so it is probably best to use a different term altogether to describe it. The (admittedly rather ugly) term, study-base, widely used in modern epidemiology, can suffice in the absence of something better. If the words 'population' and 'sample' *are* used – as inevitably they will be – then the author(s) should try to ensure that their readers understand exactly what is meant by the terms so that they are not fooled into thinking they are the real thing.

The reason that epidemiological studies on assemblages of human remains is problematic is that we have no control over the selection of these assemblages because of a number of what one might call extrinsic and intrinsic factors, to which we now give some attention.

Extrinsic Factors

The aim of a palaeoepidemiological study is to make some general statements about the characteristics of a group of skeletons based on observations made about what is usually a subset of the group as a whole, the whole group comprising all those who were buried at the site over a certain period. It is another matter, however, as to how accurately either group of dead individuals – the small or the large – reflects the reality of the living population of which it once formed a part; we shall return to this issue later.[9]

There are four extrinsic factors that act on the dead assemblage, extrinsic in the sense that they are independent of any biological features of the assemblage. They all tend to reduce the size of the study-base so that the final number of individuals (or skeletons) for study becomes smaller, and most likely, very much smaller than it was originally.

The four factors are (1) the proportion of all those who died who are buried at the site being studied, (2) the proportion of those buried whose remains survive to discovery, (3) the proportion discovered, and (4) the total recovered. The four subgroups involved are represented diagrammatically in Figure 2.1.[10] The proportional size of the original dead population lost at each stage ($p1 - p4$) varies one from the other in a manner that certainly is not constant and is not likely to be known, or, in most cases, is not even susceptible to reasonable estimatation.

The Proportion of the Dead Buried at the Site.　　There is little randomness about the place in which one is buried, this being determined by place of domicile, religious beliefs, and social mores, among other factors; some people may have chosen their place and mode of disposal in advance. A burial assemblage, therefore, is socially or culturally, not biologically, determined and to that extent might not be typical of the population of which it was once a part.[11]

The proportion of the total number of dead individuals buried at a single spot is thus affected by many different influences, and estimates of this proportion are likely to be based on guesswork rather than anything more certain. There are some exceptions, of course: at some sites the number buried may include all those who died in a battle,[12] or in a shipwreck,[13] or following some catastrophe, but such sites are generally few and far between.

Proportion Lost Owing to Disturbance and Poor Preservation.
Bodies buried in a cemetery are rarely left undisturbed for long, as is apparent to anyone who has excavated them. This is especially the case in towns where the press of people and their insatiable demand for space result in an intense pressure on the accommodations provided for predecessors.[14] There is plentiful historical evidence for this, particularly for the medieval period, when it was customary to remove bones from the ground to an ossuary to make way for the

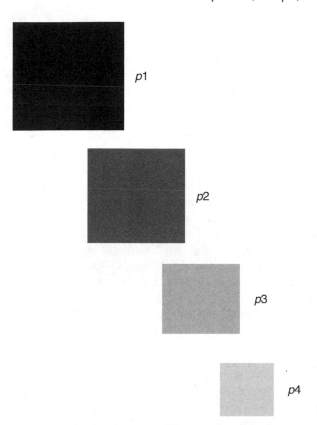

Figure 2.1 Diagram showing how losses in skeleton numbers occur at different stages; $p1$ = the proportion of those dying who are buried at the site being studied; $p2$ = the proportion of those buried who survive to discovery; $p3$ = the proportion discovered; and $p4$ = the total recovered. The magnitude of the loss at each stage will vary one from the other in a manner that will not be constant

more recent dead. Disturbance of graves can readily be confirmed by studying the site plans of any cemetery dig, where grave-cuts are obvious even to the most cursory examiner. The fully articulated, gleaming white skeleton exists only in the minds of writers of fiction; in Northern Europe at least, the reality is quite likely to be something that resembles well-chewed digestive biscuit and that may be about as easy to deal with.

The factors that govern decomposition and skeletonisation and the subsequent preservation of the skeleton have been studied, especially by forensic scientists to whom these matters are of particular interest, but they are still not fully understood.[15] The rate of decomposition is dependent on many factors and is generally quickest in dry, aerobic conditions. In optimum circumstances, a body may be skeletonised in four to six months,[16] but following burial skeletonisation almost always takes much longer.[17]

Taphonomy, that is, the events leading to the disruption and loss of skeletal elements, has been most thoroughly studied by animal bone specialists. These specialists have generally confirmed the classic study of Brain, who showed that small bones are most likely to disappear from an animal carcass together with the cartilaginous ends of long bones and that hard, dense bones survive well, often because they defeat the efforts of dogs and other carnivores to chew them.[18]

The taphonomy of human bone has not been studied with anything like the same enthusiasm, although it is known that the survival of human bone is very variable. Dense bones such as the petrous temporal or the mandible survive relatively well, as do bones with a high proportion of cortical bone. By contrast, bones with a large amount of trabecular bone do not generally survive well, and the small bones of the hands and the feet are also likely to be underrepresented, largely because they are easily overlooked during excavation.[19]

The net result of the processes of taphonomy and human activity in the graveyard is that many skeletons are found in a somewhat bedraggled state with parts missing. This situation can have unfortunate consequences when an attempt is made to decide which diseases were present, particularly some of the joint diseases, which require the presence of the small bones of the hands and the feet to facilitate diagnosis. In other cases, the burial may be represented merely by a coffin stain, all of what Todd optimistically called 'the indissoluble bone'[20] having dissolved to nothing.

The Proportion Discovered.   Where they are not obliterated by them, burial grounds are often obscured by modern civil engineers and, it must be said, by less modern ones; the enlargement of churches and cathedrals, for example, frequently encroached on graves adjacent to earlier walls. The archaeologist is able to recover only those burials that are within the power of his trowel (or earthmover) to uncover, and this proportion is subject to considerable variation and may not be constant over time, even at one site. For example, a site might have a number of well-defined phases, but the proportion of skeletons recovered of those buried during each phase can vary considerably and is likely to be completely unknown. What is more likely to be known, however, from a survey of the site, or from trial excavations or from documentary sources, is the total extent of the cemetery, as well as the proportion that has been excavated. It can thus be possible to make an estimate of the likely maximum occupancy of the cemetery, an estimate that may not be much more than a single order of magnitude in error.

Proportion Excavated.   This extrinsic factor should involve the least loss and ought to be the one that can be quantified reasonably accurately. There are always some skeletons that are too fragile to excavate, but at least a site diagram or a photograph can be studied from which sex and any obvious pathology might be evident. Optimally, a bone specialist (or some other competent person) is on site to examine the skeleton *in situ* so that not all the useful information is lost. There is a potential for further attenuation of numbers during washing, packing, and dispatch, but these losses should be few and discernable and ought not to further complicate an already perfectly awful situation.

Estimation of the Proportion Finally Examined.   In most cases it is not possible to estimate the proportion of those buried at a site who eventually come to be examined unless there are records of the numbers buried. From the site of the redundant church of St Peter's in Barton-on-Humber a total of 2,750 inhumations was recovered, dating from *ca* 950 to 1850. The parish records of St Peter's were extant from October 1566 to December 1857, from which it was found that the mean number of burials per year was about 25. Based on estimates of the population of the parish, about 11,000 bodies entered the ground at St Peter's, of which only about a quarter was recovered.[21]

Intrinsic Factors

The only intrinsic factor that needs to be considered in the present context is this: we are dealing of necessity with a dead assemblage rather than a living population. This fact may seem so blindingly obvious that it does not need saying, but it is surprisingly often overlooked, and the assemblage is treated, or referred to, as though it *is* the living population. Dead assemblages differ in some important respects from living populations, particularly in respect to their

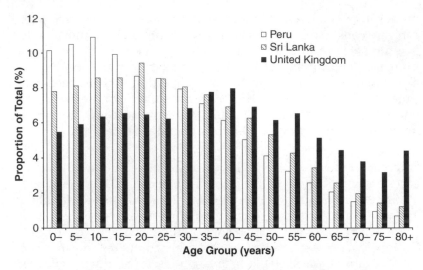

Figure 2.2   Percentage age distribution of living populations from Peru, Sri Lanka, and the United Kingdom for 2000. Note that the proportion of young people decreases and the number of the elderly increases as a country becomes more developed

age-structure. Moreover, they differ according to the stage of economic development of their country of origin.

Figure 2.2 shows the demographic profile of three contemporary living populations from countries in various stages of development. In each case there is a high proportion of young people in the population, but the proportion of older people increases with increasing development. The age distribution of a dead assemblage (Figure 2.3) in a developing country is typically U-shaped with a lot of deaths occurring at both extremes of the age range. The effect of an improving economy is to reduce the number of deaths that occur among the young, especially by reducing the infant mortality rate, so that eventually the distribution is skewed markedly to the right, as seen for the United Kingdom in the figure.

Archaeological assemblages are not exactly comparable to any modern society, but we could expect their demographic features to be much more like those of an underdeveloped or developing country, so that the age distribution of the assemblage approximates them much more closely than that of the contemporary United Kingdom.

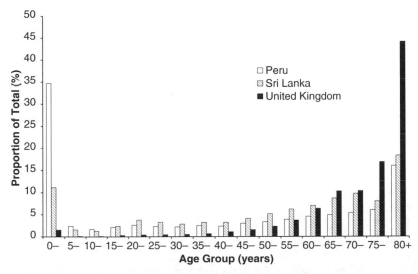

Figure 2.3   Percentage age distribution of total number of deaths in
Peru, Sri Lanka and the United Kingdom for 2000. In an
undeveloped country (Peru in this example) the distribution
is more or less U-shaped, with most deaths occurring at the
two extremes of life. As the country becomes increasingly
developed, the number of deaths in infancy and childhood
decreases, and in a fully developed country the distribution
is skewed markedly to the right, with very few deaths
before the age of 45

Time Scales

While discussing the differences between archaeological assemblages and the populations with which modern epidemiologists generally choose to work, one must mention time scales. In modern epidemiological studies, time scales are generally reckoned in decades at most; a big follow-up study of a sample designed to measure the incidence of a disease might operate over 30 years (although the study would be carried out in considerably less time using techniques described in Chapter 4). But this is about the upper end of the range; most studies operate over much shorter periods. The study-base available to the palaeoepidemiologist, by contrast, may – and usually does – represent individuals who died many hundreds of years apart, and although good phasing may be able to divide the group into subunits with shorter time periods, 100 or 200 years is

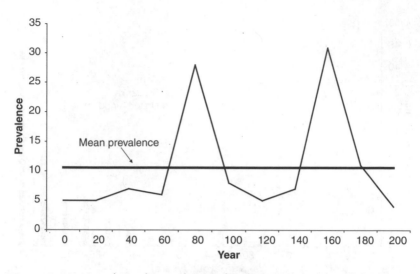

Figure 2.4 Hypothetical prevalence of a disease over time. There are two greatly increased peaks of prevalence, which tend to elevate the mean prevalence above that which is usually experienced. In a palaeoepidemiological study, these peaks will go unnoticed, and it will be impossible to correct their influence on the mean. If the converse were the case, that is, if there were periods when the prevalence was unusually low, then this would – of course – tend to give an incorrectly low estimate of the prevalence for most of the period

about as short an interval as is likely to be achieved. There are some exceptions whereby the date of death can be much more precisely known, or in which the deaths are known to have taken place over a short time – plague pits, crypt burials, and battle cemeteries are examples – but none of these is common.

The extended time scale with which one has, of necessity, to work has the effect of smoothing out differences within and between groups, as illustrated in Figure 2.4. In this hypothetical example, there are two episodes of a markedly increased prevalence of a disease over a comparatively short time, which we might assume were due to the operation of some environmental factor; because the data are studied for the entire period, these two interesting features are obscured. The overall effect is to produce a mean prevalence for the period (10.7) that is higher than that experienced by the population over the entire period, with the exception of the two crisis periods and one other toward the end of the period, which is fractionally greater than the mean. Were the position to be reversed, that is, had there been periods when the prevalence was substantially lower than usual, the net effect would have been to *reduce* the mean. There is no *a priori* means of knowing whether the prevalence in an assemblage is higher or lower than its 'real' value and so no way to correct the observed rate.

Thus in palaeoepidemiology we are dealing with a study-base that has suffered and died from diseases that are largely nonrandom, that is a social or cultural and not a biological construct, and that has suffered from a number of depredations in the time between burial and recovery. Most modern epidemiologists would at this stage be regretting ever turning their attention away from such simple matters as trying to trace cohorts of workers from factory records or arguing away negative results; the palaeoepidemiologist, however, has no choice but to proceed, because he or she is not going to get anything better to work on.[22]

In a more encouraging tone, however, we note that some checks and balances can be made to try to ensure that the study-base is in not too bad a shape. For example, the age- and sex-structures of a skeletal assemblage can be determined to see whether it fits expectations; that is, is the distribution analogous to the knowledge of the stage of development at the time? Most preindustrial societies are likely to have an age distribution that is more or less U-shaped, with a substantial number of juveniles, usually up to 30% of the total. If this is not the case, then, unless there are good reasons for this – for example, the infants were buried somewhere else, as in the Romano-British period – one should think hard before carrying out any extensive epidemiological studies on the assemblage.

The sex ratio of the adults can also be checked; this should not vary much from unity without a good reason, which is best known beforehand. For example, late Romano-British assemblages frequently have an excess of males, but the explanation for this is unclear (Table 2.1).[23]

When the sex ratio is markedly different from expected, the first uncharitable thought might be that some mistake has been made, unless the palaeoepidemiologist has also undertaken the routine anthropology. If the assemblage cannot be reexamined, however, it might be sensible to move on to more promising material.[24]

Sample Sizes

A question frequently asked of epidemiologists and statisticians, often by students but also by others who ought to know better, is this:

Table 2.1 Percentage distribution of male and female deaths at some Romano-British cemeteries

Site	Male	Female	Male:Female Ratio	N
Ilchester	63	27	2.3	43
Queensford Mill	40	60	0.7	57
Cassington	66	34	1.9	64
West Tenter Street	68	32	2.1	84
Victoria Road	61	39	1.6	85
Dunstable	53	47	1.1	86
Ashton	70	30	2.3	166
Lankhills	61	39	1.6	183
Trentholme Drive	80	20	4.0	266
Cirencester	69	31	2.2	293
Butt Road	57	43	1.3	299
The Querns	71	29	2.4	345
Poundbury	46	54	0.9	804

N = total number assigned a sex in the assemblage

Data from several sources

'Is the sample large enough?' The answer to this question can be only 'Large enough for what?' Some samples will never be large enough to provide an adequate demographic profile – 10 bodies could provide no useful information, for example, whereas 100 might, and 10 samples of 10 from closely related sites might also do so. In this case, a plot of the data would quickly show whether the result is more or less in accord with *a priori* expectations, and common sense (a commodity not to be scorned in the interpretation of data) would dictate the weight to be given to the data.

There is no magic number above which a sample becomes 'large enough', but it is possible to calculate the number needed in some circumstances. For example, suppose one wished to know how many adult skeletons should be measured to obtain a reasonable estimate of the population mean for some parameter; one could use the formula

$$n = \left(\frac{Z_\alpha \times s}{d} \right)^2$$

where n = the number of subjects required; Z_α = the probability that estimate will include the population parameter; s = the standard deviation of the parameter, and d = the tolerance within which the parameter is to be estimated.

The probability is generally fixed at 95%, in which case $Z_\alpha = 1.96$ (from t-tables); d is arrived at on the basis of an arbitrary decision; s, however, poses a problem unless it is known from other studies. If the parameter to be estimated were the mean height of the population, it is very likely that previous work would have produced results that could be used. Let us suppose we know from other studies that the standard deviation (s) of this measure is 8.0 cm for medieval males. Further, let us suppose we wish the estimated mean to be ±5 cm of the population mean; n is then simply derived as follows:

$$n = \left(1.96 \times \frac{8.0}{5} \right)^2 \approx 10.$$

This is a surprisingly small number. If, however, we wish for greater precision, the number rapidly increases. Thus for $d = 2$, $n = 62$; for $d = 1$, $n = 246$, and for $d = 0.5$, $n = 983$.

Sample size is also critical when trying to measure differences between groups as one might do, for example, in a case-control study, but again there is a formula that will supply the answer provided that some key bits of information can be fed into it. We will leave further reference to this matter until Chapter 7 and now proceed to the next area of difficulty, the definition of outcome variables.

Endnotes

1. Even though in some studies, individuals are pursued until their death, they always start the study alive.

2. L. L. Gluud, 'Bias in clinical intervention research', *American Journal of Epidemiology* 163 (2006): 493–501.

3. These matters are considered further in Chapter 9.

4. Sometimes the population is sufficiently small that all its members can be studied. This might be the case in a cross-sectional study of a group of workers in a factory, for example, although this raises another question – that is, to what extent is this group (of painters, say) representative of painters as a whole? This question need not be pursued here; those who are anxious to know more about it, and particularly about the problem of the so-called 'healthy worker effect', should consult a standard text, such as R. R. Monson, *Occupational Epidemiology*, 2nd ed. (Boca Raton: CRC, 1990).

5. Most computer programs produce numbers that are actually 'pseudo-random'. Lehmer, whose algorithms are frequently used to generate random numbers, describes a series of random numbers as 'a vague notion embodying the idea of a sequence in which each term is unpredictable to the uninitiated and whose digits pass a certain number of tests, traditional with statisticians and depending somewhat on the use to which the sequence is put' [D. H. Lehmer, 'Mathematical Methods in Large-Scale Computing Units', *Annals of the Computational Laboratories of Harvard*

University 26 (1951): 141–46]. The mathematician John von Neumann said that, 'Anyone who considers arithmetical methods of producing random digits is, of course, in a state of sin' [quoted in H. H. Goldstine, *The Computer from Pascal to von Neumann* (Princeton: Princeton University Press, 1972), p. 297].

6. For sources of bias that may follow inappropriate selection see, for example, W. Kalsbeek and G. Heiss, 'Building Bridges between Populations and Samples in Epidemiological Studies', *Annual Review of Public Health* 21 (2000); 147–69; M. Blettner, C. Heuer, and O. Razum, 'Critical Reading of Epidemiological Papers: A Guide', *European Journal of Public Health* 11 (2001): 97–101; G. R. Williamson, 'Misrepresenting Random Sampling?' *Journal of Advanced Nursing* 44 (2003): 278–88. This is not a problem confined to human epidemiology; veterinary epidemiologists are equally troubled by it [F. J. Coonraths, C. Staubach, and K. Tackmann, 'Statistics and Sample Design in Epidemiological Studies of *Echinococcus mutilocularis* in Fox Populations', *Acta Tropica* 85 (2003): 183–89].

7. M. Ganguli, M. E. Lytle, M. D. Reynolds, and H. H. Dodge, 'Random versus Volunteer Selection for a Community-Based Study', *The Journals of Gerontology, Series A, Science and Medical Sciences* 53 (1998): 39–46.

8. Of course it is perfectly possible to draw a random sample from a skeletal assemblage; however, no one should be deceived into thinking that this does anything to offset any bias inherent in the parent assemblage or that the results of the study are somehow purified by the process.

9. See Chapter 4.

10. A similar scheme with respect to assemblages of animal bones has been discussed by T. J. Ringrose ['Bone Counts and Statistics: A Critique', *Journal of Archaeological Science* 20 (1993): 121–57].

11. This point can be exemplified by considering a community with a mix of people of different national origins or religions. The individuals buried in the Methodist, Moslem, Jewish, or secular cemeteries is most unlikely to be typical of the population as a whole. With an increasing number of individual choosing to be cremated and their ashes scattered, we are almost certainly increasing the difficulties of any future palaeoepidemiologists.

12. A small number of the 28,000 individuals killed in the Battle of Towton in 1461 was recovered and found to have horrific injuries, especially concentrated around the forearms and the head. Details are plentifully supplied in V. Fiorato, A. Boylston, and C. Knüsel, *Blood Red Roses: The Archaeology of a Mass Grave from the Battle of Towton AD 1461* (Oxford: Oxbow, 2000).

13. The *Mary Rose*, Henry VIII's flag ship, went down on 19 July 1545 with an estimated 415 crew on board of whom only about 30 survived. When the ship was raised in 1982, the remains of 179 (*ca* 46% of those who drowned) were recovered. See A. J. Stirland, *Raising the Dead: The Skeleton Crew of King Henry VIII's Great Ship, the* Mary Rose (Chichester: John Wiley and Sons, 2000).

14. Further details are to be found in C. Gittings, *Death, Burial and the Individual in Early Modern England* (London: Routledge, 1984), especially Chapter 5. Ruth Richardson quotes the *Commons Journal* for 1746–1747 as saying of two London churchyards that they 'are so full of Corps, that it is difficult to dig a Grave without digging up some parts of the Corps before decayed . . .' [*Death, Dissection and the Destitute* (London: Penguin Group, 1988), p. 79].

15. One of the earliest investigators in this field was the pathologist A. K. Mant, whose research formed the basis for his MD Thesis (*A Study in Exhumation*), which was presented to the University of London in 1950. Much more recently, William Bass established the body farm at the University of Tennessee, where bodies are left in various environments to study those factors that affect decomposition. The body farm achieved a good deal of public interest through the efforts of the crime writer, Patricia Cornwell. Bass has published a general account of his own: W. J. Bass and J. Jefferson, *Death's Acre* (New York: G. P. Putnam's Sons, 2003).

16. A. Galloway, W. H. Birkby, A. M. Jones, T. E. Henry, and B. O. Parks, 'Decay Rates of Human Remains in an Arid Environment', *Journal of Forensic Science* 34 (1989): 607–16; D. A. Komar, 'Decay Rates in a Cold Climate Region: A Review of Cases Involving Advanced Decomposition from the Medical Examiner's Office in Edmonton, Alberta', *Journal of Forensic Science* 43 (1998): 57–61.

17. More information about these matters can be found in B. B. Dent, S. L. Forbes, and B. H. Stuart, 'Review of Human Decomposition Processes in Soil', *Environmental Geology* 45 (2004): 576–85; K. V. Iverson, *Death to Dust: What Happens to Dead Bodies?* 2nd ed. (Tucson, AZ: Galen Press, 2001); W. U. Spitz, *Spitz and Fisher's Medicolegal Investigation of Death: Guidelines for the Application of Pathology to Investigation*, 4th ed. (Springfield, IL: C. C. Thomas, 2006), especially Section III.

18. C. K. Brain, *The Hunters or the Hunted? An Introduction to African Cave Taphonomy* (Chicago: University of Chicago Press, 1981). There is an excellent bibliography of taphonomy to be found at *www.geocities.com/abeisaw/taphonomy.html*, and new studies appear in the *Journal of Taphonomy*, first published in 2003. Taphonomy is equally important to forensic scientists, and their needs are catered to in W. D. Haglund and M. H. Sorg, *Forensic Taphonomy: The Postmortem Fate of Human Remains* (Boca Raton, LA: CRC, 1997).

19. T. Waldron, 'The Relative Survival of the Human Skeleton: Implications for Palaeopathology', in *Approaches to Archaeology and Forensic Science*, eds. A. Boddington, A. N. Garland, and R. C. Janaway (Manchester: Manchester University Press, 1987), pp. 55–64; S. M. Bello, A. Thomann, M. Signoli, O. Dutour, and P. Andrews, 'Age and Sex Bias in the Reconstruction of Past Population Structures', *American Journal of Physical Anthropology* 129 (2006): 24–38.

20. T. W. Todd, 'Skeletal Records of Mortality', *Scientific Monthly* 24 (1927): 482.

21. T. Waldron, *The Human Remains from St Peter's Church, Barton-on-Humber*, in press.

22. One of my professors of epidemiology had a maxim: if a thing was worth doing, it was worth doing badly. Palaeoepidemiologists may gain some comfort from this.

23. At Cirencester, Calvin Wells suggested that the large excess of males that was found (approximately 2:1) was because the town was 'largely given over to retired legionaries. . . many of whom lacked regular wives and whose sexual partners, if any, were probably drawn from the professional prostitutes who were no doubt an abundant and plentiful amenity of the town'. Regrettably, none of this delightful speculation can be verified. ['The Human Burials', in *Romano-British Cemeteries at Cirencester*, eds. A. McWhirr, L. Viner, and C. Wells (Cirencester: Cirencester Excavation Committee, 1982), p. 135]. See also T. G. Parkin, *Demography and Roman Society* (Baltimore, MD: Johns Hopkins University Press, 1992).

24. It must be recognised that some material may be so important that epidemiological or statistical niceties will be of secondary (or even of no) consideration. There are

very few archaeologists who would discount an assemblage of Mesolithic skeletons on numerical grounds, and palaeontologists are used to seeing 1s and 2s as quite large numbers, even to the point of defining new species from such numbers. Frequently there is an inverse relationship between the number of subjects and the number of investigators. For example, the excavation of 28 American soldiers at Fort Erie in Canada was worked on by a team of 19 [*Snake Hill: An Investigation of a Military Cemetery from the War of 1812*, eds. S. Pfeiffer and R. F. Willikamson (Hamilton: Durn Press, 1991), whereas the number who have been called in to examine the so-called Ice Man (Ötzi) has probably broken all records. The following references give just a hint of what has been done and by whom: H. Seidler, W. Bernhard, M. Teschler-Nicola, W. Platzer, D. zur Nedden, R. Henn, A. Oberhauser, and T. Sjovold, 'Some Anthropological Aspects of the prehistoric Tyrolean Ice Man, *Science* 258 (1992): 1867–868; O. Handt, M. Richards, M. Trommsdorff, C. Kilger, J. Simanainen, O. Georgiev, K. Bauer, A. Stone, R. Hedges, W. Schaffner, G. Utermann, B. Sykes, and S. Pääbo, 'Molecular Genetic Analysis of the Tyrolean Ice Man', *Science* 264 (1994): 1775–778; M. W. Hess, G. Klima, K. Pfaller, K. H. Kunzel, and O. Gaber, 'Histological Investigations on the Tyrolean Ice Man', *American Journal of Physical Anthropology* 106 (1998): 521–32; F. Rollo, M. Ubaldi, L. Eermini, and I. Marota, 'Ötzi's Last Meals: DNA Analysis of the Intestinal Content of the Neolithic Glacier Mummy from the Alps', *Proceedings of the National Academy of Science* 99 (2002): 12594–99. There must soon be no more that the poor corpse can reveal [D. Sharp, 'Time to Leave Ötzi Alone?' *The Lancet* 360 (2002): 1530].

3 | Outcome Variables

I said earlier that epidemiology was the study of disease in populations and so it is, but epidemiologists may study other characteristics of populations. In a simple descriptive study, for example, the distribution of height, weight, or blood pressure might be determined, perhaps relating the findings to earlier studies, to look for trends over time, which are often reported as being detrimental to health – the current fascination with obesity being a good example.[1] In a so-called experimental study, the effect of reducing exposure to a toxic substance in the workplace on, let's say, reaction time in solvent workers may be examined, while the effects of a new broncho-dilator on the lung function of patients with asthma would be of interest to chest physicians. In all cases, what is being studied is often referred to as an outcome variable, or outcome measure, which is the subject of this chapter.

In palaeoepidemiology the number of outcome variables that can be studied is limited by the nature of the material; of those that are available, disease is the most significant.

Disease

Before the frequency of disease in a skeletal assemblage can be determined there must be ways of recognising the diseases that are present and of giving them names that will enable others to recognise them also; in other words, they need to be classified in some way. This classification is usually referred to as a diagnosis.

The Purpose of Diagnosis in Clinical Practice

Diagnosis is one of the three bases of clinical practice, the two others being prognosis and treatment. The purpose of diagnosis has always been to allow the physician to give a prognosis to his patient and to suggest possible forms of treatment. So far as we can tell, the manner of arriving at a diagnosis has changed very little throughout the course of medical history. First the physician elicits signs and symptoms presented by the patient; at some periods the physician might supplement these with some direct observations, either of the patient or one of his or her bodily fluids; until comparatively recently, the only fluid available for examination was the urine. Having got together as much information as possible, the physician then constructs a differential diagnosis in which all the conditions that might conceivably give rise to some, or all the signs and symptoms, are mentally or actually tabulated. The intellectual task that then follows is to arrange the differential diagnoses in an order of probability and so arrive at the disease that is most likely the one from which the patient is suffering.[2] Having made this decision, the physician informs the patient of the likely outcome and the extent to which it might be affected by treatment. The importance of the physician arriving at the correct diagnosis does not need emphasising since it could make the difference between treatment and no treatment, perhaps between life and death. The antiquity of this procedure is attested to by the Edwin Smith papyrus, which is thought to have been written around 1600 BCE.[3] In this document the physician is instructed how to make the diagnosis, which is to be relayed to the patient in one of three ways: as

An ailment which I will treat;
An ailment with which I will contend; or
An ailment not to be treated.

Nothing much has changed in the intervening four or five thousand years except that the patient is now almost always examined, investigations have become vastly more complex, and there have been important changes in treatment. Until about 50 years ago remedies were generally ineffective but harmless; now, some at least have become very effective but also potentially very harmful.

On occasion the physician is not satisfied with a primary diagnosis and, instead, may seek a secondary one. For example, the diagnosis of gout depends on demonstrating a number of signs and symptoms but especially a raised blood uric acid concentration. This may be due to an inability to excrete uric acid in the urine (so-called primary gout), but it may be due to a number of secondary causes. The diagnosis of gout, therefore, may not be sufficient in itself to allow treatment to begin; this may have to wait for the secondary diagnosis. There are many other instances in which this would be the case.

The Nature of Diagnosis

To the lay mind, diagnosis has the air of a precise – if not an exact – science, but hardly anything could be further from the truth. The vocabulary of diagnosis is actually rather confused and imprecise and incorporates many different features or attributes of the patient's condition. Thus a diagnosis may simply be a symptom (biliary colic), a sign (jaundice), a description of a pathological organ (mitral stenosis), a clinical measurement (hypertension), an abnormal radiological appearance (osteopoikilocytosis), or an abnormal laboratory result (hyperlipidaemia). In fact, the way in which diseases are classified reflects the uncertainty about what it is that really constitutes a disease in the first place, and this accounts for the great variety of labels used. Some years ago Kendall elegantly summed up the position in a way that has not been bettered, as:

> rather like an old mansion which has been refurbished many times, but always without clearing out the old furniture first, so that amongst the new inflatable plastic settees and glass coffee tables are still scattered a few old Tudor stools, Jacobean dressers and Regency commodes, and a great deal of Victoriana.[4]

As Scadding and his colleagues suggested many years ago, it is probably a lack of logical cohesion in our definition of individual diseases that has resulted in us being unable to produce a satisfactory definition of disease as a whole.[5] One substantial bar to progress is that doctors are very little interested in what one might call the philosophy of disease, because for the purposes of the practice of medicine, the name given to the disease does not matter so long as it conveys what the doctor needs to know about the likely outcome and the direction treatment should take. A diagnosis can be taken as a piece of shorthand for saying something like, 'this is the disease that will linger on and may get much worse unless I treat it with such and such a medicine'. We might call this disease 'lobar pneumonia' but just as easily 'the lung disease that we treat with ampicillin'. The second description lacks a certain finesse, however, and might have to be modified somewhat to differentiate it from other lung diseases that are treated with the same or other antibiotics.

Changing Fashions in Diagnosis

One of the difficulties that face those who are interested in the history of medicine, and particularly those who wish to detect temporal trends in disease, is that it is hard to compare like with like. Descriptions of symptoms may be inadequate and, except in the last few decades, are extremely unlikely to be supplemented with any of the information that is so necessary nowadays for making a diagnosis, especially the results of laboratory tests or radiography. Moreover, the original author will have assumed that his reader well understood what he meant by 'rachisagra' and, on this account, would not have bothered to go into too much detail about it; but for those who come upon his work several decades, or several centuries later, the meaning may be completely incomprehensible.[6] There is also an irresistible tendency among doctors to engage in 'splitting', that is, to render what once appeared to be one disease into several parts. This can be well illustrated by a consideration of the joint diseases.

Among the very early medical writers no distinction was drawn between any of the diseases that affect the joints; osteoarthritis, gout, rheumatoid arthritis, rheumatic fever, and the others were all thought to be part of a single entity and generally referred to as gout. This state of affairs continued until the late sixteenth century, when Guillaume de Baillou (1538–1616) made the distinction between gout and rheumatic fever and the other forms of joint disease. Baillou was also the first to use the word *rheumatism* in anything like its modern sense. The distinction between gout and other arthropathies was made very explicitly by Thomas Sydenham (1624–1689), writing in the middle of the seventeenth century; his description of the pain as being like a dog gnawing one's foot is one with which modern sufferers will feel much sympathy. William Cullen's (1710–1790) description of rheumatism in the eighteenth century was notable for dividing the symptoms into those that were acute and affected the joints and muscles and those that were chronic and affected only the joints. This distinction was also maintained by Charles Scudamore (1779–1849) who, in 1827, published the first systematic treatise of rheumatism in English.[7]

Rheumatoid arthritis had probably been recognised as different from other forms of joint disease in the seventeenth and eighteenth centuries, but priority for the first clinical description is generally given to Augustin Landrè-Beauvais (1772–1840), who worked at the Salpêtrière in Paris; in his MD thesis of 1800 he referred to it as *goutte asthénique primitive*, thus preserving the notion that it is a form of gout.[8] The concept of infectious arthritis was first suggested by Charles-Joseph Bouchard (1837–1915), who noted that the joints were involved in many infectious diseases; he coined the term *pseudo-rheumatisme infectieux* for them and divided them into those in which the organism was known and those in which it was not. The association between urethritis, especially of gonoccocal origin, and joint disease was well recognised during the eighteenth century, which was something of a golden age for venereal disease but was rediscovered by Hans Reiter (1881–1969) in the early twentieth century, when he described it in a German soldier, since when it has been called Reiter's syndrome.[9]

The first accurate descriptions of ankylosing spondylitis were published during the later years of the nineteenth century and are particularly associated with the names of Pierre Marie (1853–1940) and Ernst Adolf von Strümpel (1853–1925). It was not until 1904, however, that it was clearly differentiated from other forms of spondyloarthropathy.

The first complete clinical account of osteoarthritis was given in 1829 by Léon Cruveilhier (1791–1874), who described the osteophytes seen around the joint as arising *ex morbo rheumatico*. During the later part of the nineteenth century, accounts of osteoarthritis appeared in many countries and by many authors, including Rudolf Virchow (1821–1902), who is generally considered to have been the first to use the term *arthritis deformans* for this condition.[10] So by the beginning of the twentieth century, a number of separate conditions were known to affect the joints, some of which were subdivided into acute and chronic forms. Acute rheumatism was generally taken to mean only rheumatic fever, whereas among the chronic forms were osteoarthritis, gout, rheumatoid arthritis, and some forms of infectious arthropathy.

The most significant trend in recent times has been the recognition of the sero-negative arthropathies. Before the 1950s it was thought that rheumatoid arthritis was a nonspecific syndrome that might be triggered by a number of different aetiological factors such as psoriasis, urethritis, and ulcerative colitis. During the 1950s these variants of classical rheumatoid arthritis came to be seen as discrete entities, and this view was strengthened by the demonstration that the serum of those with these disorders did not contain a particular immunoglobulin that was found in patients with classical rheumatoid arthritis and that came to be known as rheumatoid factor;[11] the conditions in which rheumatoid factor was absent thus came to be known as the sero-negative arthropathies.

Two things emerge from studying the history of joint – or indeed, any other – disease. Firstly – and obviously – understanding the nature of the disease depends on notions of aetiology that prevailed at the time. Before the discovery of microorganisms, for example, the notion of infection as a cause of joint disease was not possible; similarly, before the development of immunology, the idea of a sero-negative arthropathy was unimaginable and is nowhere to be found in texts written before about the mid-1960s.[12]

Secondly, changing fashions in diagnosis often make it extremely difficult to render diagnoses made in former times into their modern equivalents. This difficulty is compounded by the plethora of terms that may be used for the same condition. For example, osteoarthritis may be referred to in early writings as arthritis deformans, senile arthritis, morbus coxae senilis, or as spondylitis deformans;[13] nowadays the term *osteoarthrosis* is sometimes used as an alternative to osteoarthritis to escape the connotations of inflammation implied by the ending '-itis', and some writers persist with the use of the old-fashioned *degenerative joint disease*. Ankylosing spondylitis may be found masquerading under the names of Marie-Strümpel disease, Bechterew's disease, bamboo spine, poker back, pelvospondylitis ossificans, rheumatismal ossifying pelvospondylitis, spondyloarthritis ankylopoietica, atrophic ligamentous spondylitis, ossifying ligamentous spondylitis, rhizomelic spondylitis, and, confusingly, spondylitis deformans. I dare not go on with any further examples, but you see the problem.

Those who read the early medical literature, therefore, must learn not always to give modern meanings to the diagnoses in these sources. Thus when Wood Jones writes in 1908 of the skeletons from Nubia that 'the disease which shows itself with by far the greatest frequency... is rheumatoid arthritis',[14] we might express considerable surprise unless we realise that he is actually referring to what we would now call osteoarthritis and not rheumatoid arthritis, in which case we have no reason to disagree with him. It is not surprising, therefore, that some modern palaeopathologists take the view that the only way to know what was meant by diagnoses in the old literature is to reexamine the bones themselves, if indeed they are still available for study.

Making a Diagnosis

Clinicians rely on three sources of information to make a diagnosis: the patient's history, which among other things will tell them what symptoms the patient has; the clinical examination from which they will elicit a number of signs; and a range of supplementary examinations that will include laboratory tests, radiography, and pathology. The diagnosis may sometimes be made on the basis of the patient's history alone, or it might be made only after the most exhausting series of supplementary examinations – and it is the patient who is usually most exhausted at the end of them. Clinicians also use the information obtained to follow a diagnostic algorithm, although they may be unaware that this is what they are actually doing, since the steps through the sequence may be taken unconsciously. However the diagnosis is done, the aim is to find the most parsimonious explanation for the data at hand.

Conventionally, medical students are taught to construct a differential diagnosis, that is, a list of *all* the diseases that might conceivably account for the patient's condition. These are then structured in such a way that they come to be arranged in order of probability, the first on the list being the most probable and – by inference – the one with which the patient is afflicted. In practice, this long-winded approach is frequently circumvented except during formal case presentations, when it is incumbent on the presenter to outdo the audience in finding the most rare conditions to include in the differential diagnosis.

For some diseases, criteria have been developed that must be satisfied before a diagnosis can be made. Those for the spondylarthropathies are shown in Table 3.1.[15] Of the nine criteria shown,

Table 3.1   Criteria for diagnosing spondylarthropathies[a]

Inflammatory spinal pain or synovitis, plus at least *one* of the following:
Positive family history
Psoriasis
Inflammatory bowel disease
Urethritis
Acute diarrhoea
Alternating buttock pain
Enthesopathy
Sacroiliitis

[a]Based on Dougados et al. (1991)

only two, enthesopathy and sacroiliitis, are at all amenable to demonstration in skeletal material. And this, of course, is the problem when one attempts to make a diagnosis on skeletal material that relies on clinical criteria; there is simply too little information – few signs, no symptoms, no soft tissues to examine (except possibly in the case of mummified bodies, and these are the exception rather than the rule), and a rather limited set of supplementary examinations. And when one remembers that, in an average rheumatology clinic perhaps a quarter of the patients never receive a definitive diagnosis, some doubts must be raised about the wisdom of trying to do it all on dry bones. On the bright side, however, those who examine human remains do have a few advantages over their clinical colleagues, and these will be mentioned later.

The Accuracy of Diagnosis

Those with no experience of diagnosing disease in the living often have an exaggerated idea of its accuracy; there is a common view that diagnostic compartments are completely separate entities and that every constellation of signs and symptoms fits into one, and only one, box. This is akin to thinking of diseases as occupying a unique space in what one might consider as a diagnostic diagram, by analogy with a number diagram in which every number can be located by reference to two coordinates (the number 2i, 5, for example, has a unique position shared by no other number). The truth is generally otherwise, however; the boundaries between diseases (even between health and disease) are frequently blurred and may overlap. Pathological processes are dynamic, progressing, relapsing, and the final nature of a patient's disease may not be known until several weeks or months after it has first been declared. In a substantial proportion of cases, a diagnosis is never made, or a euphemism is applied, both to appease the patients who gain some reassurance by the fact that their doctors seem to know what is ailing them and to save the doctors the embarrassment of having to admit that they do not know what it is.

Having made a diagnosis, what are the chances of it being correct? Regrettably, not very high, certainly not as high as the medical profession would wish their patients to believe. Several studies have been made of the accuracy of clinical diagnosis, and they confirm what all doctors knew but were reluctant to admit. A review of 53 studies in which antemortem diagnoses were compared with autopsy findings showed that in 42, the primary cause of death was wrongly diagnosed (major error), whereas in 37, errors were made by the clinician that might have affected the outcome (class I errors).[16] The median major error rate was 23.5% (range 4.1–49.8%); the median class I error rate was 9.0% (range 0 – 20.7%). These results do not make comfortable reading, but despite this, autopsy rates are everywhere falling.[17]

Making a Diagnosis of Disease in Human Remains

When making a diagnosis from human remains, one almost always relies on the gross appearances of any abnormalities present, or – in a relatively few instances – on radiology. This is a sadly small list compared with the information in the hands of the clinicians, who, as we have seen, are not that good at diagnosis even then. And not only are most of the vital pieces of evidence that might be supplied to the clinician by the patient missing, the disease is entirely static, so that there is no possibility of waiting to see how it might develop; the appearances are those present at one particularly unfortunate moment for the individual, the time of death.

A small number of conditions that affect the skeleton have pathognomonic signs, and it is now possible to confirm some diagnoses by immunological methods or by extracting the DNA of pathogens from bone, but the opportunities to do this are limited.[18] We have seen that clinical criteria may not always be apposite to diagnosis in human remains, and the same is true of some radiological criteria, so those wishing to diagnose disease in human remains must perforce have recourse to other means of diagnosis; the most useful one in this context is a well-tried epidemiological ploy, the use of operational definitions.

Operational Definitions

'Diagnosis is by far the greatest problem [in palaeopathology]' Don Brothwell commented ruefully in 1961, and little has happened in the last 50 years or so to change this view.[19] It should be apparent by now that those who study disease in human remains are very unlikely to outshine their clinical colleagues in diagnostic acumen, and their chances of being able to make fine distinctions between different clinical entities must be reckoned somewhat slim. In many cases the most that can be achieved is a broad classification of lesions, and lumping, rather than splitting, should be the norm.[20]

If the results of studies of human remains cannot be directly compared they have little value, except perhaps to the investigators themselves, and those who report such studies should always refer to the criteria used to make their diagnoses, or at least to the published source that they have used, just to give other investigators a chance. The use of operational definitions, which may well vary – and vary widely – from clinical criteria, will have the advantage that diagnoses will be standardised and will be directly comparable among studies.

Attempts have been made to produce operational definitions for some of the joint diseases and infectious diseases. In the case of osteoarthritis, the condition can be safely diagnosed by the presence of eburnation on the joint surface, since this is pathognomonic of osteoarthritis[21]; and although we suggested using minor criteria when eburnation is not present,[22] it is much more reliable to base the diagnosis solely on the presence of eburnation, since it is a sign that ought not to be missed. If other conditions have pathognomonic signs, then this makes the diagnosis easy and – in effect – these signs *are* the operational definition.[23] In the absence of pathognomonic signs the operational definition must, of course, have clinical validity and not be based on personal preference or prejudice. Table 3.2 shows an operational definition for rheumatoid arthritis that relies mostly on observational criteria supplemented to some extent by radiology, since, as with the diagnosis of the other erosive arthropathies, the clinical classification relies to a large extent on signs and symptoms that cannot be determined from the skeleton.

For an operational definition to be useful it must be able to reject both false-positive and false-negative cases. If the true prevalence of a condition is P, then

$$P = P_{od} - P_p + P_n$$

where P_{od} = prevalence determined using the operational definition;
P_p = number of false positives; and
P_n = number of false negatives.

Table 3.2 Operational definition of rheumatoid arthritis[a]

Presence of symmetrical, marginal erosions affecting small joints of hands and/or feet
No significant new bone proliferation
Sacroiliac joints spared
Absence of spinal fusion

[a]Note that all four criteria *must* be present for the definition to be applied. Other, nonessential signs may also be noted in affected skeletons, including osteopaenia around affected joints, bony ankylosis, especially of the wrist, and eburnation of affected joints.

Table 3.3 Sensitivity and specificity

		Operational Definition	
		Negative	Positive
Disease	Absent	a	b
	Present	c	d

Sensitivity = $d/(c + d)$. This is also known as the true positive rate.
Specificity = $a/(a + b)$. This is also known as the true negative rate.

The efficacy of the operational definition can be determined by calculating its sensitivity and specificity. The sensitivity determines the proportion of cases with the disease correctly diagnosed by the operational definition – the specificity, the proportion of cases *without* the disease that is correctly rejected by it. The method of determining sensitivity and specificity is shown in Table 3.3; a good operational definition will have a high sensitivity and a high specificity, that is, will have few false positives or false negatives.

In the ideal situation,

$$P_{od} = P,$$

but, in practice this is seldom the case; the true prevalence is almost always likely to be underestimated.

It is obviously a major undertaking to make operational definitions for all the diseases of the skeleton, but if this is not done, then palaeopathology and palaeoepidemiology are likely to sink into chaos, and the possibility of making sensible deductions from published data will become more and more remote. The undertaking is not made any the less awesome by the fact that the definitions will have to be acceptable to at least the majority of those working in the field; they will have to be universally used, and any changes made in the light of increasing (clinical) knowledge will similarly have to be generally agreed on. What is really needed is for palaeoepidemiologists and/or palaeopathologists (usually one and the same) to produce a volume analogous to *DSM IV-TR*;[24] in this way the procedure for arriving at a diagnosis in human remains will become less like trying to navigate through a minefield with the aid of the sun and a Mickey Mouse watch.

Precision and Accuracy in Measuring Outcome Variables

The study of outcome variables is palaeoepidemiology is often used for comparative purposes or to test specific hypotheses: Does mean height vary between an urban and a rural assemblage; is there a difference in the distribution of joint disease over time; are spondylolysis and spina bifida occulta likely to occur together in the same individual? Whatever the purpose of the study, however, care must be taken that the determination of the outcome variable is precise, accurate, and free from bias. The precision of a set of observations is a measure of their reproducibility, and their accuracy is the degree to which they reflect the true value of the observations. Good precision does not necessarily mean the measurements are accurate, however; this point is frequently explained by reference to target shooting. Close grouping of shots at the periphery of a target may indicate good precision but poor accuracy, whereas a tight cluster in the bull indicates good precision *and* good accuracy. Bias, as already explained, refers to systematic error that distorts the outcome.[25]

Precision can be increased by ensuring that any equipment to be used is reliable and calibrated if necessary. Better precision would be achieved by measuring the length of a long bone with a measuring board that incorporates a steel rule from which the length can be read directly rather than by using graph paper from which the exact length has to be estimated. The reproducibility of results should always be determined before carrying out a study by measuring intraobserver error; when a number of observers are to be used in a study, then some measure of interobserver error should also be made. To do this, conduct observations on a sample of material that need not be taken from the study material. For example, in a study of changes in height over time, use the maximum length of the femur as the basis of the estimation. Before measuring the study material, do repeat measurements on femurs that might be obtained from another study or that constitute part of a teaching collection. Record the lengths and next day repeat the measurements, preferably not in the same order. Assessing the agreement between the two measurements can be carried out most simply by plotting them on a graph to see how far they deviate from perfect agreement, represented on the graph as a line at 45° to each axis. This would quickly and easily show any gross discrepancies. More formally, one could calculate the kappa (κ) statistic. Kappa is a number varying from 0–1 indicating none, or perfect, agreement between two sets of observations; in an intraobserver study one would hope for excellent agreement with $\kappa > 0.8$.[26]

Interobserver errors can be assessed in a similar way, again using κ as a measure of agreement. Where there is a considerable degree of error of either kind, the cause must be investigated and rectified, and the main study should not start until a satisfactory level of agreement is achieved. If this seems an overly elaborate or even an unnecessary step to take, be assured that large intra- and interobserver errors have been found in standard anthropological and dental measurements, and in recording cranial nonmetric traits.[27]

Measurement Scales

Measurement scales are widely used in epidemiology and may also be used in palaeoepidemiology for such things as grading degrees of calculus on teeth, osteophyte formation, and dental traits. In determining the age or sex of a skeleton, the scales may consist of a number of items that are scored separately and summed to give an overall 'maleness' or 'femaleness' score, for example.

There are four kinds of measurement scale: nominal, ordinal, interval, and ratio.

- Nominal scales simply assign items to groups or categories – sex, or race, for example – and on this account are sometimes also known as categorical scales.
- An ordinal scale is a numerical scale in which higher numbers represent higher values, but the intervals are not necessarily equal.[28] On a scale measuring the degree of alveolar disease in a jaw, for example, a rating of 3 indicates greater change than one of 2 but may not represent the same difference as exists between a rating of 3 and one of 4. There is no true zero point in an ordinal scale; the lowest value is arbitrarily fixed and may be any number to suit the observer.[29]
- In an interval scale, the difference between units is the same across the entire range of the scale, but again there is no true zero, so it is impossible to say how many times higher one reading is than another. The Fahrenheit scale of temperature is a good example of an interval scale; equal differences in the scale represent equal differences in temperature, but a temperature of 40° is not twice as warm as one of 20°.
- The ratio scale is similar to the interval scale but does have a true zero. An example is the measurement of height, which has a true zero value and where a measurement of 160 cm is twice as great as one of 80 cm.

When analysing data obtained using measurement scales, use the appropriate statistics. A mean can be calculated for interval and ratio scales, whereas for nominal scales the correct measure of central tendency is the mode. There is some debate about the correct statistic to use for ordinal scales; most statisticians would say that the median should be used because the intervals on the scale are not equal,[30] but, despite this, the mean is very frequently calculated and reported.

Most scales used in palaeoepidemiology are likely to be ordinal (where direct measurements are not made), and they are often used as a measure of the severity of a disease or of the magnitude of expression of a particular trait. As an example of the first, one might consider the changes in a joint with osteoarthritis; the second might be ranking the size of a Carabelli cusp on a molar. For such scales to have any meaning, they should have some clinical or other validity; for example, there should be evidence that the value given to the changes around a joint correlate with the symptoms experienced by a patient or with the progression of the disease, since this is what is understood clinically by severity. Or, is there evidence that a large Carabelli cusp has more significance than a small one, or is it simply presence/absence that matters? Unless there are some sound reasons for using measurement scales, they are best avoided; when authors insist on their use, editors or examiners should ask for justification.

Rating Scales

Rating scales are used in epidemiology to measure quantities that cannot be measured explicitly; they are extensively used in psychiatric epidemiology to measure anxiety and depression. In palaeoepidemiology their use seems to be confined pretty much to the determination of sex and age of skeletons, and several schemes have been proposed.[31] The scale will consist of a number of items that must measure the same thing and also be internally consistent. A useful statistic for measuring the internal consistency of a rating scale is Cronbach's alpha (α)[32] – see Table 3.4 – and those who devise new scales should ensure that there is internal consistency by calculating α before using them in earnest.

Table 3.4 Formula for calculating Cronbach's alpha

$$\alpha = \frac{k}{k-1}\left(1 - \frac{\sum s_i^2}{s_T^2}\right)$$

where k = number of items
s_i^2 = variance of the ith item
s_T^2 = variance of the total score formed by summing all the items

Endnotes

1. See, for example V. J. Lawrence and P. G. Kopelman, 'Medical Consequences of Obesity', *Clinics in Dermatology* 4 (2004): 296–302. Jutel, by contrast, presents the view that the risks of obesity have been exaggerated [A. Jutel, 'Does Size Really Matter? Weight and Values in Public Health', *Perspectives in Biology and Medicine* 44 (2001): 283–26].

2. Those unable to shake off a Bayesian tendency will recognise this as a Bayesian approach: the physician is arranging possible diagnoses in the light of prior probabilities and adjusting prior probabilities as the consultation proceeds [C. J. Gill, L. Sabin, and C. H. Schmid, 'Why Clinicians Are Natural Bayesians', *British Medical Journal* 330 (2005): 1080–83]. Physicians are by no means the only medical practitioners to seize the Bayesian initiative; surgeons [S. M. Alvarez, B. A. Poelstra, and R. S. Burd, 'Evaluation of a Bayesian Decision Network for Diagnosing Pyloric Stenosis', *Journal of Paediatric Surgery* 41 (2006): 155–61] and radiologists [E. S. Burnside, 'Bayesian Networks: A Computer-Assisted Diagnosis Support in Radiology', *Academic Radiology* 12 (2005): 422–30) are also jumping on the band wagon, but it is clear that by no means all are using the technique correctly [G. J. van der Wilt, M. Rovers, H. Straatman, S. van der Bij, P. van den Broek, and G. Zielhuis, 'Policy Relevance of Bayesian Statistics Overestimated?' *International Journal of Technological Assessment in Health Care* 20 (2004): 488–92], and there is no suggestion 'that the bayesian approach is a perfect means of reaching a correct diagnosis' (Gill et al., p. 1083). As we shall see, nor is any other method.

3. Breasted's account of the papyrus is probably still the best [J. H. Breasted, *The Edwin Smith Surgical Papyrus* (Chicago: Chicago University Press, 1930)]. The text can be viewed at *www.touregypt.net/edwinsmithsurgical.htm*.

4. R. E. Kendall, *The Role of Diagnosis in Psychiatry* (Oxford: Blackwell, 1975), p. 20. Kendall also discusses the concept of disease and gives other references to this difficult area. Since Kendall wrote, more modern furniture has been placed within the old mansion to complement the plastic settees and glass tables; it too will – no doubt – soon be as outdated as the rest.

5. E. J. Campbell, J. G. Scadding, and R. S. Roberts, 'The Concept of Disease', *British Medical Journal* 2 (1979): 757–62. The debate continues, the majority of authors tending toward the rather obvious view that disease is the opposite of health [P. D. Toon, 'Defining "Disease" – Classification Must Be Distinguished from Evaluation', *Journal of Medical Ethics* 7 (1991): 197–201]; J. Bircher, 'Towards a Dynamic Definition of Health and Disease', *Medicine, Health Care and Philosophy* 8 (2005): 335–41), which begs the question of what is meant by 'health' [J. Kovacs, 'The Concept of Health and Disease', *Medicine, Health Care and Philosophy* 1 (1998): 31–9]. It is clear that we are still far from having a satisfactory notion of either health or disease [see, K. Sadegh-Zadeh, 'Fuzzy Health, Illness, and Disease', *Journal of Medical Philosophy* 25 (2000): 605–38; L. Nordenfelt, 'On the Place of Fuzzy Health in Medical Theory, *Journal of Medical Philosophy* 25 (2000): 639–49].

6. For those who *may* not know, this is an archaic word for backache.

7. C. Scudamore, *A Treatise on the Nature and Cause of Rheumatism with Observations on Rheumatic Neuralgia and on Spasmodic Neuralgia, or Tic Doloureaux* (London: Longman, Rees, Orme, Brown and Green, 1827).

8. The full title of the thesis was *Doit-on admettre une nouvelle espèce de goutte sous la denomination de goutte asthénique primitive*. The text of the thesis has been reproduced in 'The First Description of Rheumatoid Arthritis'. Unabridged thesis of the doctoral dissertation presented in 1800, *Joint Bone Spine* 68 (2001): 130–43. Those who have presented MD or other theses in recent years will be amazed at the size of this one.

9. The French (who like to do things their own way) prefer to call the condition Fiessinger-Leroy disease; they described it independently of Reiter in 1916.

10. There is as yet no really comprehensive history of the joint diseases, and I have leaned heavily on R. A. Stockman's account written in 1920 (*Rheumatism and Arthritis*, Edinburgh: W. Green) for much of the information in this section. His book contains references to some of the original texts, and others are to be found in the list provided by W. S. C. Copeman in the introductory chapter to the first edition of his *Textbook of the Rheumatic Diseases* (Edinburgh: Livingstone, 1948).

11. Rheumatoid factor is one of the so-called autoantibodies produced by autoreactive B lymphocytes. These cells are normally quiescent but may become stimulated to produce autoantibodies that may have serious pathological consequences [E. A. Leadbetter, I. R. Rifkin, A. M. Hohlbaum, B. C. Beaudette, M. J. Shlomchik and A. Marshak-Rothstein, 'Chromatin-IgC Complexes Reactivate B Cells by Dual Engagement of IgM and Toll-Like Receptors', *Nature* 416 (2002): 595–98].

12. It is interesting to follow the changes in the understanding of joint diseases in the text books of rheumatology. In Copeman's book [*Textbook of the Rheumatic Diseases* (Edinburgh: Livingstone, 1948)] reference to rheumatoid factor appears first in the third (1964) edition; the first and second editions appeared in 1948 and 1955, respectively. Not until the fourth (1969) edition, however, is the nature of the rheumatoid factor 'so well established that it is no longer necessary to discuss the several arguments against it' (p. 187); it is in this edition also that the term sero-negative first appears.

13. Some of the cases referred to as spondylitis deformans in the past were probably ankylosing spondylitis rather than osteoarthritis. This can sometimes be verified from photographs of the affected spine but otherwise, this has to remain as another area of uncertainty.

14. F. Wood Jones, 'Pathological Report', in *The Archaeological Survey of Nubia, Bulletin No. 2* (Cairo: Ministry of Finance, 1908), p. 55.

15. M. Dougados, S. van der Linden, R. Juhlin, B. Huitfeldt, B. Amor, A. Calin, A. Cats, B. Dijkmans, I. Olivierieri, G. Pasero, E. Verys, and H. Zeidler, 'The European Spondylarthropathy Study Group Preliminary Criteria for the Classification of Spondylarthropathy', *Arthritis and Rheumatism* 34 (1991): 1218–27.

16. K. G. Shojania, E. C. Burton, K. M. McDonald, and L. Goldman, 'Changes in Rates of Autopsy-Detected Diagnostic Errors Over Time', *Journal of the American Medical Association* 289 (2003): 2849–56.

17. See, for example, Royal College of Pathologists of Australasia Autopsy Working Party, 'The Decline of the Hospital Autopsy: A Safety and Quality Issue for Healthcare in Australia', *Medical Journal of Australia* 180 (2004): 281–85.

18. Immunological methods have been used to diagnoses multiple myelòma by extracting the abnormal myeloma protein from bone [C. Catteneo, K. Gelsthorpe, P. Phillips, T. Waldron, J. R. Booth, and R. J. Sokol, 'Immunological Diagnosis of Multiple Myeloma in a Medieval Bone', *International Journal of Osteoarchaeology* 4 (1994): 1–2],

and the polymerase chain reaction (PCR) has been used to extract DNA of the bacteria that cause tuberculosis and leprosy [for example, see H. D. Donaghue, M. Spigelman, C. L. Greenblatt, G. Lev-Maor, G. K. Bar-Gal, C. Metheson, K. Vernon, A. G. Nerhlich, and A. R. Zinc, 'Tuberculosis: From Prehistory to Robert Koch, as Revealed by Ancient DNA', *The Lancet Infectious Diseases* 4 (2004): 584–92; R. Montiel, C. Garcia, M. P. Canadas, A. Isidro, J. M. Guijo, and A. Malgosa, 'DNA sequences of *Mycobacterium leprae* Recovered from Ancient Bones', *FEMS Microbiological Letters* 226 (2003): 413–14; H. D. Donaghue, A. Marcsik, C. Matheson, K. Vernon, E. Nuorala, J. E. Molto, C. L. Greenblatt, and M. Spigelman, 'Co-Infection of *Mycobacterium tuberculosis* and *Mycobacterium leprae* in Human Archaeological Samples: A Possible Explanation for the Historical Decline of Leprosy', *Proceedings, Biological Sciences Royal Society* 272 (2005): 389–34]. Both immunology and PCR can be used only to *confirm* a diagnosis; a negative result will not necessarily lead to the diagnosis being rejected since one cannot detect a false-negative result. In the case of a DNA analysis, false-negative results may be due to the fact that DNA is present in very small amounts and is often extensively degraded; however, false-positive results may readily be caused by contamination with modern DNA [D. Mitchell, E. Willersley, and A. Hansen, 'Damage and Repair of Ancient DNA', *Mutation Research* 571 (2005): 265–76].

19. D. Brothwell, 'The Palaeopathology of Early Man: An Essay on the Problems of Diagnosis and Analysis, *Journal of the Royal Anthropological Institute* 91 (1961): 318–44.

20. Lumping is the process of grouping entities into broad categories. For example, psoriatic arthropathy, Reiter's syndrome, and rheumatoid arthritis can all be lumped together under the rubric of erosive arthropathies; very often it will not be possible to define erosive changes seen in the skeleton beyond this broad category.

21. This is not *strictly* true since in other joint diseases in which the articular cartilage is destroyed (such as rheumatoid arthritis) eburnation may develop; there should be no difficulty in differentiating these conditions from osteoarthritis, however.

22. J. Rogers and T. Waldron, *A Field Guide to Joint Disease in Archaeology* (Chichester: John Wiley & Sons, 1995), p. 43ff.

23. Other skeletal conditions with pathognomonic signs include spondylolysis, osteomyelitis, and both syphilis and leprosy when the full-blown lesions in the skull are present.

24. *Diagnostic and Statistical Manual of Mental Disorders,* 4th ed. (text revision) (New York: American Psychiatric Association, 2000). The manual provides operational definitions for all recognised psychiatric disorders.

25. Mathematically it can be shown that the bias (B) and precision (P) can be equated to accuracy (A) as follows: $A^2 = B^2 + P^2$. Thus if bias can be reduced to zero, accuracy and precision are equal.

26. J. R. Landis and G. G. Koch, 'The Measurement of Observer Agreement for Categorical Data', *Biometrics* 33 (1977): 159–74.

27. M. Kouchi, M. Mochimaru, K. Tsuzuki, and T. Yokoi, 'Interobserver Errors in Anthropometry', *Journal of Human Ergology* 28 (1999): 15–24; C. J. Utermohle and S. L. Zegura, 'Intra- and Interobserver Error in Craniometry: A Cautionary Tale', *American Journal of Physical Anthropology* 57 (1982): 303–10; J. A. Kieser and H. T. Groeneveld, 'The Reliability of Human Odontometric Data', *Journal of the Dental Association of South Africa* 46 (1991): 267–70; J. E. Molto, 'The Assessment and

Meaning of Intraobserver Error in Population-Based Studies Based on Discontinuous Cranial Traits', *American Journal of Physical Anthropology* 51 (1979): 333–44.

28. These are also often known as ranking scales.

29. In an ordinal scale, numbers need not be used at all, but the intervals can be indicated by letter, A, B, C and so on; the same constraints apply as when numbers are used, of course.

30. See, for example, S. Siegel and N. J. Castellan, *Nonparametric Statistics for the Behavioral Sciences*, 2nd ed. (New York: McGraw-Hill, 1988), pp. 25–8.

31. See, for example, J. E. Buikstra and D. H. Ubelaker, *Standards for Data Collection from Human Skeletal Remains*, Research Series No. 44 (Fayetteville, AR: Archaeological Survey, 1994).

32. J. M. Bland and D. G. Altman, 'Cronbach's Alpha', *British Journal of Medicine* 314 (1997): 572.

4 | Measures of Disease Frequency

The most commonly used measures of disease frequency are incidence and prevalence. The incidence (or incidence rate) of a disease is most simply defined as the number of new cases that occur in a population at risk over a certain period of time:

$$I = \frac{\text{number of new cases}}{\text{population at risk}} \text{ per unit time}$$

where I = the incidence.

This definition is reasonable so long as the population at risk remains relatively constant over the study period, which it may do when one is estimating incidence over short periods. Over longer periods, by contrast, the population may change by virtue of births, deaths, and migrations, and modern epidemiologists now more frequently relate the incidence to person years at risk, which is calculated by totaling the time during which each member of the population was at risk; this period at risk, of course, ends when the person contracts the disease under study (or dies). In this case:

$$I = \frac{\text{number of new cases}}{\text{total years at risk}}$$

Prevalence, by contrast, is a simple proportion and is calculated simply as:

$$P = \frac{\text{number of cases}}{\text{total population}}$$

where P = the prevalence.

Prevalence has no time base, and so it is not a true rate although it is very frequently referred to as such. Note that the denominators for calculating incidence and prevalence are different and may often be very different, particularly when one is studying a disease with a high prevalence.

Relationship between Incidence and Prevalence

Each individual who newly contracts a disease is an incident case and enters the prevalence pool where he or she remains until recovery or death. If recovery and death rates are both low, then the relationship between incidence and prevalence approximates to:

$$P = I \times D$$

where I = incidence, P = prevalence, and D = the average duration of the disease.

Where the average duration is short, as with many of the common infections of childhood, P and I may be similar. Where the average duration is long, P may be many times greater than I, and this is the case with chronic diseases such as osteoarthritis.[1]

Epidemiological Methods for Measuring Incidence and Prevalence

Incidence

The determination of an incidence rate requires a period of observation, which may be short or long depending on the natural history of the disease. The procedure involves defining a population to study, frequently referred to as a cohort, and then following it up carefully and counting the number of new cases of the disease in question that occur during the follow-up period. For example, the population might be all the school children in a London borough who are followed up for a period of 3 months to determine how many contract chicken pox, having first excluded all those either with, or who have had the disease, at the start of the study period since they cannot, by definition, be at risk of contracting it again.[2] This type of study is usually known as a prospective,[3] follow-up, or cohort study.

The design of a study to measure the incidence of an infectious disease is about as simple and straightforward as anything can be in epidemiology. But consider the investigator who wishes to study the induction of bladder cancer in men who may have been exposed to chemicals in making dyes. He or she will establish a study population that might be all the men currently working in the appropriate industries and will probably stipulate that all should have a minimum period of exposure before being entered into the study – which might be 6 months or a year – to eliminate those with very slight exposure. The only task that remains is to sit back and count the number of new cases of bladder cancer as they arise. A colleague, however, mentions that bladder cancer may take up to 20 or 30 years to develop, and, since there are very few investigators who are prepared to wait so long for their results, and fewer grant-giving bodies prepared to fund such a study, a way round this dilemma must be devised. The trick in such a study is to define what is known as an historical cohort and follow it up over a long period that also ends some time in the past. For the dye workers example, the cohort might be established as all those working in the industry on, say, 1 January 1950, and the follow-up period might end on 31 December 1989, 40 years later. Cases that arise during the follow-up period will form the numerator in the calculation, and the total number of person years at risk will form the denominator.[4] This type of study may be called a retrospective prospective study, or an historical cohort study.

Relative Risk

A follow-up study can also be used to estimate the risk of exposure to perceived hazards, be they exposures in the work place, personal habits, or the taking of prescription drugs. The actual form of the study varies according to the circumstances, but consider a factory where some workers are exposed to a dust thought to give rise to a disease of the lungs. Two cohorts might be established, one with exposure to the dust and one without, and the number of cases that occurs in both groups could be determined over the study period. Assume that the results were as shown in Table 4.1: then the risk of contracting the lung disease in those exposed is 72/2054; in those without exposure it is 16/3078. The *relative risk* (sometimes also known as the risk ratio) is thus:

$$\frac{72/2054}{16/3078} = \frac{72 \times 3078}{16 \times 2054} = 6.96 \ (95\% \ CI \ 4.06 - 11.90)^5$$

where 95% CI = 95% confidence interval.

Table 4.1   Results of hypothetical study of dust exposure and lung disease

	Lung Disease		
	Yes	No	Total
Exposed	72	1982	2054
Not exposed	16	3062	3078
Total	88	5044	5132

Relative risks in excess of 2.0 are usually thought of as being worthy of attention, so in our hypothetical case, the risk of the exposure is considerable.[6]

Prevalence

Prevalence is measured using what is referred to as a cross-sectional study. In this type of study, a population is defined and the number of individuals found to have the disease of interest within it are counted. The prevalence is then simply the number with the disease divided by the number in the study population. If one were interested in the prevalence of back pain in office workers, for example, the result would almost certainly differ depending on when the study was carried out, since the number of individuals with and without back pain might be expected to vary from time to time, just as the number of fat globules in the salami will depend on where you slice it. Suppose that on one occasion the number of office workers was 487 and a simple questionnaire showed that the number with back ache was 63; then the prevalence = 63/487 = 129.4 per thousand. As with the relative risk – or indeed any other epidemiological measure – it is more satisfactory to report the prevalence with a 95% confidence interval, which is this case is 102.4 – 162.1. Let us suppose the study is repeated 3 months later. We then find that 473 employees are in the office, and our questionnaire shows that only 48 report having back pain. The prevalence is now 101.5 per thousand (95% CI 77.4 – 132.0%). Are we to conclude that things in the office have improved? There is no significant difference between the prevalence on the two occasions (since the confidence intervals overlap), and the most likely explanation is that – if anything – things may have got worse and that some of those with backache are now in such pain that that they cannot attend for work.[7]

Point and Period Prevalence

A distinction is sometimes made between point prevalence and period prevalence, depending on whether the observations are made once, or several times over a period and averaged out; point prevalence (from a single observation) will tend to underestimate the true prevalence.[8] This distinction has little relevance to palaeoepidemiologists, however, since there is only one chance to make an estimation, albeit usually over a long time period. Every epidemiological study on human remains is, thus, a cross-sectional study.[9]

Crude and Age-Specific Incidence and Prevalence

When calculated using the whole study population as the denominator, the incidence and prevalence so obtained are known as *crude* rates. This is not generally a useful measure; it is more usual to calculate age- and sex-specific rates by breaking the population into different age groups for each sex and calculating the rates for each in turn. These rates are essential for comparative purposes, as will be discussed in the next chapter.

A Note on Teeth

Dental diseases are common in most assemblages of human remains and include dental caries, teeth lost antemortem, abscesses, and periodontal disease. There are some special problems associated with recording the prevalence of caries and missing teeth that need to be mentioned.

In modern dental epidemiology, the frequency of dental disease in the permanent teeth is determined using the *DMFT* index, which records the number of caried teeth (*D*), the number missing as a result of caries (*M*), the number filled (*F*), and the total number examined (*T*).[10] The index in each subject is calculated by adding *D*, *M*, and *F* and dividing by *T*. For populations, the mean index is usually quoted, although other indices have been suggested.[11] When examining milk teeth, the *deft* index is used, where *e* refers to teeth extracted because of caries and the remaining initials are the same for the index applied to the permanent teeth.

It is clear that the *DMFT* has rather limited application for human remains because there are no filled teeth, and it is by no means certain that all teeth that were lost antemortem were lost on account of caries. Instead, when recording caries, one usually expresses the number of caried teeth as a percentage of the total number of teeth present in the assemblage. This is not a very helpful statistic, however, firstly because the result is biased because molar teeth survive better than anterior teeth[12] do, and it is molars that are mostly affected by caries,[13] and so there is a bias toward overestimating the proportion of caried teeth. The mean caries index (DT) can, of course, be determined and expressed as a mean for that part of the assemblage with teeth extant, and the same thing can be done for missing teeth (MT), remembering that by no means all the missing teeth will have been lost through caries. The DT is a much more useful summary than simply recording the number of caried (or missing) teeth as a proportion of the total number of teeth.[14] What is more interesting clinically, however, is to know what proportion of individuals had dental disease, irrespective of the number of teeth affected, although the number of bad teeth may also be recorded and reported separately.[15]

For dental abscesses it is best simply to record the number of individuals in whom these are present and express this as a proportion of the total with teeth examined. There is nothing against recording and presenting the number of abscesses in each case if it is believed that this adds to the overall picture of dental health in the assemblage, however. For alveolar disease the simplest method is to report the proportion of individuals with alveolar bone loss that exceeds 3 mm measured from the cement-enamel junction to the crest of the alveolar margin on at least one tooth.

Other Measures of Morbidity and Mortality

There are several other measures of morbidity and mortality, some of which need briefly to be mentioned here; they include proportional mortality and a number of events relating to childbirth and early life.

Proportional Mortality Ratio

The proportional mortality ratio (PMR) expresses the ratio of the number of deaths from one cause to the total number of deaths from all causes. It may be used in modern epidemiology when there are difficulties in establishing the proper denominators to use.[16] It is also possible to calculate a proportional morbidity ratio (also usually – and confusingly – referred to as a PMR). The use of the PMR has rather fallen out of favour in modern epidemiology, other methods (described in Chapter 6) being preferred.

Adverse Effects Associated with Childbirth and Early Life

The most significant event associated with childbirth is death, either of the child or the mother, and several different measures of the death rate are used, depending who has died and when death occurred. Allusions to at least some of these rates are to be found in the palaeopathological and palaeoepidemiological literature. Those I will mention briefly are the maternal mortality rate, the stillbirth and perinatal mortality rates, and the neonatal and infant mortality rates.

Maternal Mortality Rate (MMR).   This is the ratio of maternal deaths to the number of live births in a year:

$$MMR = \frac{\text{number of maternal deaths occurring in pregnancy or within 42 days of delivery}}{\text{number of live births}}$$

and is usually expressed per 10^4 or 10^5 live births.

Stillbirth Rate (SBR).   This is the proportion of fetal deaths to the total number of live births and fetal deaths.

$$SBR = \frac{\text{number of fetal deaths occurring after 24 weeks}}{\text{number of live births} + \text{fetal deaths}}$$

and is usually expressed as 10^3 per year. The rates excludes miscarriages from the numerator, that is, losses occurring before the 24th week of gestation.[17]

Perinatal Mortality Rate (PNMR).   This expresses the number of fetal deaths occurring after 24 weeks' gestation plus deaths of infants in the first week of life as a proportion of all live births and fetal deaths of 24 weeks or more.

$$PNMR = \frac{\text{number of fetal deaths after 24 weeks} + \text{infant deaths} \geq 7 \text{ days}}{\text{number of live births} + \text{fetal deaths} \geq 24 \text{ weeks}}$$

The PNMR is generally given per 10^3 and per year.

Infant Mortality Rate (IMR).   This is the proportion of infants dying in the first year of life compared with all live births.

$$IMR = \frac{\text{number of deaths during the first year}}{\text{total number of live births}}$$

Neonatal Mortality Rate (NNMR).   This compares the number of deaths in the first 28 days of life with the number of live births.

$$NNMR = \frac{\text{number of deaths} < 28 \text{ days}}{\text{total number of live births}}$$

The IMR and NNMR are conventionally given per 10^3 per year.

Rates for Use in Palaeoepidemiology

It should be obvious from what has been said so far that incidence can *never* be measured in palaeoepidemiological studies, because neither the nominator nor the denominator can be known; there is neither means of determining *new* cases nor of knowing the magnitude of the population at risk. Because of the cross-sectional nature of all studies of disease frequency, it is point prevalence that is being measured, usually with a time base measured in decades or centuries.

Proportional morbidity ratios (but not, of course, proportional *mortality* ratios) can be used in palaeoepidemiology, although it may not always be a simple matter to define morbidity since there is no sudden change from normal to abnormal appearances in bone; we are not dealing with a dichotomous variable but rather with a sliding scale with 'normal' at one end and 'abnormal' at the other, and the decision as to when the cross-over point is reached is often a matter of opinion rather than of fact. In any study of PMRs, then, it is incumbent on the investigators clearly to define their criteria of morbidity, especially if they were hoping that other workers might be able to confirm their observations.

Since all the rates relating to childbirth have a denominator that includes the number of live births, none is appropriately used in palaeoepidemiology. The so-called stillbirth rate that is sometimes reported, in which the total number of fetal skeletons is related to the total number of children, is simply the prevalence of fetal skeletons in the assemblage. Rates that require the number of *live* births in the denominator can never be calculated in palaeoepidemiology because there is no way to determine how many children have been born to the living population from the assemblage. It may sometimes be possible to estimate the number of live births, however, if there are extant parish records that give the number of christenings in the parish, a number that can be taken as approximately equal to the number of births. For example, at St Peter's in Barton-on-Humber the parish records showed that a total of 7,359 christenings had taken place between 1570 and 1850, an average of 26 per year. The number of fetal deaths that were reliably phased to this period was 57, which was considered to be about a quarter of those actually buried there. Assuming this to be the case, then the stillbirth rate was approximately 31 per thousand, a rate that seems plausible and that is at least the same order of magnitude of those found in contemporary developing countries.[18]

Predicting Prevalence in the Living from an Assemblage of Human Remains

It is clearly of interest to know whether it is permissible to predict the frequency of diseases in a living population from the prevalence in an assemblage of human remains, since it is the characteristics of the living with which one is most concerned when trying to reconstruct past societies. In this consideration there are important differences between those diseases that do not contribute to death and those that do, and so they will be dealt with separately.

Diseases That Do Not Contribute to Death

Many of the diseases that fall into this class and that affect the skeleton are of long duration, and they are broadly of two types, those in which new cases arise only – or predominantly – in childhood or adolescence (for example, spondylolysis, and some of the skeletal dysplasias) and those in which new cases arise first during adult life and continue to do so at all subsequent ages; osteoarthritis is the prime example of this second kind of disease.

We can take spondylolysis as the model for the first type. It arises in childhood, and for the present purposes we can take it that cases do not arise thereafter.[19] The duration of the resulting lesion is for the lifetime of the individual – except with surgical intervention and this is not a consideration here – and so the prevalence of the condition increases from zero at (say) age 5 to a maximum at (say) age 20, and it remains at this rate for all subsequent ages (see Figure 4.1). With increasing age some of those with the disease will die, thus decreasing the numerator, but the total numbers in the population will also be decreasing; hence the denominator will also reduce in size, and the prevalence will, therefore, tend to remain relatively constant.

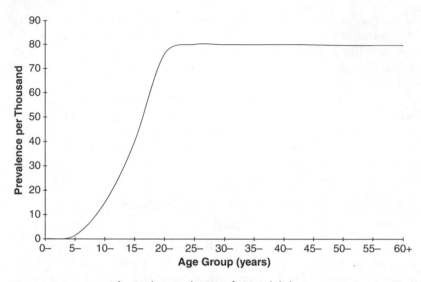

Figure 4.1 Hypothetical prevalence of spondylolysis at varying ages. The prevalence increases from zero to a maximum at age 20 and remains constant thereafter

Taking osteoarthritis as the model for the second type of disease we see a completely different natural history.[20] This disease tends to occur first in middle adult life, and the incidence increases steadily with increasing age thereafter. Because the duration of the disease is for the lifetime of the individual, the prevalence also increases steadily with age, and in extreme old age, there is scarcely anyone who has not got at least one joint affected.

In cases where the disease does not (or does not materially) contribute to death it is reasonable to suppose that the prevalence in a skeletal assemblage is a reasonable estimate of the prevalence in the living, using the same criteria for diagnosis in the two. Consider any living population in which a proportion of the adults has osteoarthritis. Since this disease will not adversely affect survival to a significant degree,[21] and it is not associated with any other condition that does, the fact of having osteoarthritis does not in itself contribute to the probability of dying, and so an individual with osteoarthritis is as likely or not to die as one without the disease. The proportion of those who die with osteoarthritis with thus be no different from the proportion of those who survive with it, and the ratio between the numerator and denominator in the living and dead will be approximately equal, even though the age structure of the two will differ, as we have seen in Chapter 2.

I can illustrate this with a simple model. Suppose we have an adult population with a prevalence of osteoarthritis of 30%. The population consists of 500 individuals, and osteoarthritis will be distributed among 150 of them by using random number tables. The whole population is then subjected to death rates ranging between 5 and 75%, those dying determined by the use of random number tables again. The prevalence of osteoarthritis among the dead is determined by counting the number who were allocated the disease in the first stage of the procedure. The estimate of the prevalence among those who die in each of five separate trials is shown in Table 4.2. The mean prevalence among the 'dead' group provides an acceptable estimate of the prevalence in the living, although it tends to be more accurate with higher death rates; the standard error of the estimate decreases with increasing death rate as would be expected. Even with a 5% death rate, however, the estimate, although low, is not significantly different from the expected 30%, and there is no significant difference between the mean of the five estimated rates ($F = 2.15$, $p > 0.05$). It is also clear from the table that the best estimate of the living prevalence is obtained from the mean of several studies.

Table 4.2 Modeled prevalence rates for osteoarthritis in a skeletal assemblage[a]

	Death Rate in Population (%)				
Trial	5	10	25	50	75
1	20.0	32.0	29.6	30.4	30.1
2	16.0	46.0	23.2	32.8	31.2
3	20.0	22.0	31.2	26.0	30.9
4	16.0	36.0	36.0	32.4	31.2
5	40.0	32.0	34.4	29.6	30.9
Mean	22.4	33.6	30.9	30.3	30.9
SD	10.0	8.6	5.0	2.7	0.5
SEM	4.9	3.9	2.2	1.2	0.2

SD = standard deviation

SEM = standard error of mean

[a]In each trial the number of individuals who die is determined by random number generation having previously allocated osteoarthritis among 150 (30%) the original group of 500, also by random number generation. The numbers in the cells show the prevalence of osteoarthritis found among the dead, assuming different death rates.

Diseases That Do Contribute to Death

When we are dealing with diseases that do contribute to death, then the prevalence in skeletal assemblages generally does not approximate to those in the living. I will illustrate this point with some modern data from South Africa, a country where tuberculosis is one of the leading causes of death and thus has some resemblance to the situation in England during the sixteenth to nineteenth centuries. The number of cases of tuberculosis reported in the last year on record (2003) was 206,110, whereas the number of deaths from this cause was 50,568, a case-fatality rate (CFR) of 24.5%.[22] Tuberculosis accounted for 11.2% of all deaths, and this could be considered the palaeoepidemiological prevalence, that is, the prevalence one might expect in a skeletal assemblage, assuming that all the cases could be accounted for. Assuming that each incident case lives on average 4 years, the prevalence in the living population of approximately 40 million is about 2%.[23] The palaeoepidemiological prevalence, therefore, is a considerable *over*estimate of that in the living. The effect of different CFRs is shown in Table 4.3, where it can be seen that the palaeoepidemiological prevalence overestimates the living prevalence until the CFR is 5% when the living prevalence is accurately predicted; with an increasing CFR the error in the estimate of the living prevalence becomes increasingly great, whereas with a CFR less than 5%, the living prevalence is *under*estimated.

That the prevalence in the living cannot be predicted from the palaeoepidemiological prevalence holds true for any killing disease, but whether there is an *under-* or an *over*estimate depends on the proportion of all deaths that is due to the disease in question, and its CFR. It will also depend crucially, on whether or not *all* the dead cases can be ascertained in the skeletal assemblage, and, unfortunately this is seldom the case. In the case of tuberculosis, for example, the propor-

Table 4.3 Effect of different case-fatality rates on apparent palaeoepidemiological prevalence of tuberculosis[a]

	Case-Fatality Rate (%)					
	25	20	15	10	5	1
Prevalence (%)	11.2	9.2	6.9	4.6	2.3	0.5

[a]Based on modern data from South Africa (www.statssa.gov.za and WHO 2005). Tuberculosis actually accounted for 11.2% of all deaths with a case fatality rate of 24.5%, and the prevalence of tuberculosis in the living population was about 2%, a figure greatly overestimated with case fatality rates in excess of 5%.

tion of cases in which the skeleton is affected seems to vary a good deal, depending on which report one reads, but it is agreed that it is only a minority and almost certainly never more than 30%.[24] This will – of course – result in the detection of fewer cases and cause further errors in the estimate of the living prevalence.

Missing Data

So far the calculations of disease frequency have been discussed as though the skeletons with which we are likely to be dealing were complete, but as everyone who has examined human bones knows, the occasions on which this is true are all too few. Small bones of the hands and the feet are often lost, and the disturbance of the grave commonly also causes damage to, or loss of, larger elements. This has an important bearing on any sums that are done to calculate prevalence. For example, suppose that we have 120 adult skeletons in 27 of which there is evidence of osteoarthritis of the spine; suppose also that a further 19 have osteoarthritis of the hands, and 4 have osteoarthritis of the hip. The crude prevalence for each would appear to be 225, 158.3, and 33.3 per thousand, respectively. But what if the spines of 17 of the skeletons were too damaged to examine, if 13 lacked hands and 9 had hips missing? How should we represent the prevalence knowing this? One way would be to present them as a range of possibilities. If we make the assumption that *none* of the missing joints was affected, then we are left with the original prevalences. However, if we assume that they were *all* affected, then we obtain rates of $(27 + 17)/0.12$, $(19 + 13)/0.12$, and $(4 + 9)/0.12$ per thousand, or 366.7, 266.7, and 108.3, respectively. These estimates can be thought of as representing the upper limit of the range and the original rates to represent the lower limit; the true rate lies somewhere between.

This is a valid but somewhat cumbersome way of going about things and would lead to fearsome problems when one is trying any comparative work. An alternative is simply to ignore the missing data, recognising that this would lead to an underestimate of the prevalence, but this is not at all satisfactory. We could also make the assumption that the distribution of osteoarthritis amongst the missing joints is similar to that in the joints that *are* present and use the number present minus the number missing as the denominator. Thus the denominators in the example given above now become 103 $(120 - 17)$ for the spine, 107 $(120 - 13)$ for the hands, and 111 $(120 - 9)$ for the hips. With these denominators, the prevalences are now 262.1, 177.6, and 36.0 per thousand, respectively; we might perhaps

Table 4.4 Different prevalence rates for osteoarthritis derived from skeletal assemblages with missing data[a]

	Prevalence per Thousand		
Site Affected	Uncorrected Crude Rate	Uncorrected Upper Rate	Corrected Rate
Spine	225.0	366.7	262.1
Hands	158.3	266.7	177.6
Hip	33.3	108.3	36.0

[a]The uncorrected crude rate assumes that none of the missing elements was affected by osteoarthritis. The uncorrected upper rate assumes that that they were *all* affected, whereas the corrected rate uses the total number of elements, minus those missing as the denominator. See text for further details.

call these the corrected prevalences. (All the figures discussed so far are shown in Table 4.4 for comparison.)

Of the three solutions outlined above, the last is to be preferred, although there is a final modification that needs to be made when only one of a pair of joints is missing from an assemblage. I can illustrate this with another hypothetical example.

Consider a group of 115 skeletons, 7 of which have osteoarthritis of the hip; the crude (uncorrected) prevalence is 7/0.115, or 60.9 per thousand. Now suppose that a total of 17 joints is missing; it might be thought that the corrected prevalence would be 7/(155 − 7), or .71.4 per thousand, but this is not necessarily so. Let us further suppose that only 4 skeletons lack both hips and that 9 lack only a single hip, with 2 showing osteoarthritis in the hip that *is* present. We now have 13 skeletons with one or more hip joints missing, but we know that two of these skeletons have osteoarthritis in at least *one* hip. The total number of skeletons for which we lack any information about the presence of osteoarthritis, therefore, is only 11. The denominator for the prevalence is thus 104 (115 − 11), and the prevalence is 7/0.104, or 67.3 per thousand. In general terms, therefore, the denominator for paired joints is the number of skeletons with both joints present plus the number of single joints (that is, *one* of the pair) that show evidence of disease.[25]

Prevalence of Multifocal Diseases

For many conditions estimation of prevalence is straightforward, but for conditions that affect more than one part of the skeleton this may not be the case. Tuberculosis and osteoarthritis are good examples, although the ways to deal with each differ. Tuberculosis may affect any part of the skeleton, although the lesions are usually solitary or affect only a single element, such as the spine,[26] whereas osteoarthritis may affect several joints in the same individual. What is usually done in such cases is to determine the prevalence by skeletal element or by separate joints using the number of extant elements or joints as the denominator. In the case of tuberculosis, or any disease that causes solitary lesions, the overall prevalence can be calculated simply by summing the prevalences for individual elements. So, if the prevalence of tuberculosis of the spine is 6 per thousand, of the hip 2 per thousand, and of the wrist 3 per thousand, then the overall prevalence is 11 per thousand.

In the case of osteoarthritis, however, the overall prevalence is *not* the sum of the prevalence for each joint, because individuals with polyarticular disease will contribute more than once. It is, in fact, rather complicated to calculate the overall prevalence, but one scheme has been proposed that relies on careful recording of all joints present and of all joints with disease.[27] The scheme is best explained by reference to Table 4.5. In this table the presence or absence of osteoarthritis has been scored for each of the joints in the skeleton ($J1 - Ji$) as being present (1) or absent (2). Where no observation can be made because the joint is missing or too badly damaged to examine, a score of zero (0) is entered. In the table, the entries are shown for a series of cases from $1 - i$. The prevalence of osteoarthritis at individual joints is calculated by summing all the entries recorded as 1 ($\Sigma 1$) in each column and all those recorded as either 1 or 2 ($\Sigma(1+2)$). The prevalence for individual joints is then simply:

$$\frac{\sum(1)}{\sum(1 + 2)}$$

In Table 4.5, there are two entries in column J1 where a 1 has been entered, there are five entries with complete information (1 or 2 being entered), whereas for the remainder of joints there is no usable information. The prevalence for J1 is, therefore, 400 per thousand.

To calculate the overall prevalence, we have to turn to the entries in the rows of the table. The numerator is the sum of the all the rows in which a 1 has been entered (the number of 1s in each row is immaterial). The denominator is the sum of the number of rows in which a 1 has been recorded, plus the entries that have a complete

Table 4.5 Hypothetical data for presence or absence of osteoarthritis in different joints in a skeletal assemblage[a]

Case No.	J1	J2	J3	J4	J5	J6	—	Ji	No. of Cases with Positive Score	No. of Cases with Complete Observations
1	1	1	2	2	1	2	—	2	1	1
2	2	2	2	2	2	2	—	2	0	1
3	1	2	2	2	2	2	—	0	1	0
4	2	0	0	0	0	0	—	0	0	0
5	0	1	2	2	1	2	—	2	1	0
6	0	0	0	0	1	2	—	0	1	0
i	2´	2	2	2	2	2	—	2	—	1
Σ(1)	2	2	0	0	3	0	—	0	0	1
Σ(1+2)	5	5	5	5	6	6	—	4	4	3

[a]J1 – Ji refer to different joints in the same individual (case number 1 – i). The presence of osteoarthritis is denoted by a 1 in the row or column; the absence of osteoarthritis is denoted by a 2; where there are missing data, a 0 is inserted. Where the presence of osteoarthritis is a case is positive, a 1 is shown in column 11. Where a case has a complete set of observations (1 or 2 in each column) a 1 is shown in column 12. At the foot of column 11 the total number of cases with osteoarthritis is shown, while at the foot of column 12, the number of cases with complete observations is shown. The denominator for calculating the prevalence is the sum of the these numbers; the numerator is the number of cases with osteoarthritis irrespective of the number of joints affected. The table is modified from that shown in Law (2005).

set of 2s. The formula for the calculation is as above. In the table, four rows contain a 1 and three more contain complete information (a full set of 1s + 2s); these totals are shown at the foot of columns 11 and 12. The overall prevalence, therefore, is 3/7 = 430 per thousand.

This method can, of course, be used to calculate the overall prevalence of any multifocal disease where the prevalence is not the sum of the prevalence for individual sites.

Disarticulated Material

It is by no means unusual that investigations of human remains are carried out on assemblages that consist of a jumbled mass of bones coming from an unknown number of individuals. Faced with such an assemblage, one customarily calculates a minimum number of individuals (MNI) on the basis of the most frequent anatomical element present. This figure cannot be used as a denominator for calculating prevalence, however, It *is* permissible to use the number of each type of bone or joint as the denominator in the calculation, and the number of diseased bones or joints as the numerator, although there generally is little value in doing so since there is no means of knowing how representative this jumbled mass is of the original burial assemblage, nor can we be sure that individuals do not appear more than once in either the numerator or the denominator.

Further Implications for Palaeoepidemiology

What remains in this chapter is to discuss the implications of the topics so far mentioned for the interpretation of data obtained from the examination of human remains. There are three areas to consider: the nature of the diseases or conditions present in the assemblage; the establishment of *a priori* assumptions against which to test the data; and, lastly, dealing with missing data.

The Nature of Diseases or Conditions. The prevalence of disease in a skeletal assemblage will probably be a reasonable estimate of the prevalence in the corresponding living population only in those diseases that do not contribute to death.[28] Thus, when making an inference about the frequency of disease in a community on the basis of the evidence in their bones, one must know into which category the disease fits. For the disease that occurs most commonly in the skeleton – osteoarthritis – there is not much difficulty, although there are marginal problems. The old woman who is confined to bed with an arthritic hip or knee and who is immobile is at risk of succumbing to hypostatic pneumonia, and, in some societies, those whose disease meant they could not work may not have been fed. Not much will be lost if such problems are ignored, especially since there are no solutions to them.

Most infectious diseases that affect the skeleton are likely to have shortened the expectation of life either directly or indirectly, and their prevalence in the living cannot be estimated correctly; the magnitude of the error will depend on the case-fatality rate. Unfortunately, there is little that can be done to determine this and so no means of knowing how to correct any estimate to make it more realistic.

In the case of tuberculosis, the CFR was likely to have been high until well into the middle of the nineteenth century, when the number of deaths decreased well in advance of any knowledge of the true cause of the disease and long before any effective treatments were available.[29] Leprosy, by contrast, probably did not have a high mortality rate *per se*,[30] but the associated secondary infections that follow on the loss of sensation in the feet and the hands, and the social ostracism that was the concomitant of the disease, would have made the sufferer a poor risk to any historic insurance company.

Osteomyelitis stands somewhere between tuberculosis and leprosy, epidemiologically speaking. Long survival times are compatible with the disease, but there is a possibility that the infection will spread to other organs, or give rise to septicaemia, and it may also cause death through renal failure secondary to the production of amyloid in the kidney.[31]

These few examples illustrate the need to take great care when projecting skeletal prevalence back to the living population. When comparing skeletal prevalence with modern published rates, there are more complications, both because the methods for ascertaining cases in modern epidemiological work almost always differ from the operational definitions used in palaeoepidemiology and because the populations used are different. For example, modern prevalence may be related to a random sample of the whole population, to patients attending a clinic or hospital, or to those on the list of a general practitioner. In most cases it is best to consider published modern rates and palaeoepidemiological rates as quantitatively incompatible, although they may be *qualitatively* comparable; increasing with age, higher in one sex than another, tending to occur more frequently in one skeletal element than another, and so on. Quantitative comparisons are best reserved for other groups of skeletons.

A priori *Assumptions*.   A knowledge of the natural history of the diseases to be found in the skeleton permits palaeoepidemiologists to generate some *a priori* assumptions against which to test their data. To take a simple case; in any group of adult skeletons, no matter what their provenance, osteoarthritis will be the most common disease. If this is *not* the case then the group must be unusual in some respect, perhaps because it has an overrepresentation of young adults. Two constant features of osteoarthritis are that its prevalence increases steadily with increasing age and that the disease is slightly more common in women (especially elderly women) than in men. Consequently, if these features are not reflected in the skeletal group under examination, it must be unusual in some way. If the expected increase in prevalence with age is not found, then this may be because the estimation of the ages of the skeletons is inaccurate and might indicate that the task should be undertaken again by another observer. It goes without saying that the signs of osteoarthritis (or indeed any other disease) should never be used as ageing criteria, for if they are, age-specific prevalences cannot be estimated, and comparison with other studies becomes impossible.

A priori assumptions can be made about other diseases, and palaeoepidemiologists should try to devise as many as possible to apply to any study group. If the number of skeletons is too small to allow for valid inferences about these assumptions, then it will certainly be too small to allow for any epidemiological inferences, no matter how much statistical legerdemain is indulged in, and it would be best to go on to something else, or wait until further data are to hand.

Missing Data.   Missing parts bedevil the examination of human remains, and it is almost axiomatic that the skeletons that appear to have the most interesting pathology will be in the most dire condition. To deal with the problem of incomplete skeletons, one must record the number of separate elements of the skeleton (including, of course, the teeth) and the number of joints, and not merely the number of individuals, since the latter will scarcely, if ever, be used as the denominator for calculating prevalence. It would be nice to think that authors would tell their readers how they dealt with the problem of missing data and, preferably, what denominators were used to calculate the prevalence of each disease. If this would make the text too tedious to read, the information could be consigned to an appendix, or perhaps available from the author on request; it would be best to make very strenuous efforts not to put it on microfiche, since this is most certain way I know of ensuring that it would never again see the light of day.

Endnotes

1. This is a somewhat simplified account of incidence and prevalence. Epidemiologists seem to like nothing more than making simple things complicated, and those who might wish for mathematical derivations should consult K. J. Rothman and S. Greenland, *Modern Epidemiology*, 2nd ed. (Philadelphia: Lippincott Williams & Wilkins, 1998), especially Chapter 3.

2. This is not quite true, since it *is* possible to contract chicken pox twice, although rather uncommon. It should be noted also that some epidemiologists would say that any infection is a *new* infection regardless of whether or not the individual has had it before. As a general principle, however, those with the disease, or who have previously had it, are excluded from the denominator in an incidence study.

3. The term 'prospective' applied to a follow-up study seems to have been coined by Richard Doll and Austin Bradford Hill in their classic study of doctors and smoking: 'The Mortality of Doctors in Relation to Their Smoking Habits', *British Medical Journal* i (1954): 1451–55.

4. For a recent study of bladder cancer in dye workers see K. D. Rosenman and M. J. Reilly, 'Cancer Mortality and Incidence among a Cohort of Benzidine and Dichlorodenzidine Dye Manufacturing Workers', *American Journal of Industrial Medicine* 46 (2004): 505–12.

5. The 95% confidence interval represent the limits that will contain the true relative risk on 95% of all occasions. The method for determining confidence intervals for this and other measures, together with a handy computer program, is to be found in D. G. Altman, D. Machin, T. N. Bryant, and M. J. Gardner, *Statistics with Confidence*, 2nd ed. (London: British Medical Association, 2000).

6. It is very important to distinguish between *relative risk* and *absolute risk*. In my hypothetical example, the absolute risk of contracting lung disease for the exposed group is approximately 35 per thousand, so that, the high relative risk notwithstanding, the great majority of those exposed to the dust do *not* contract the disease. We will return to this point again in Chapter 8.

7. Although a hypothetical account, this example illustrates the need in a modern prevalence study to enquire about those members of a potential study group who are absent; in most instances the result of absentees will be to underestimate the true prevalence.

8. For the reason given in the previous footnote.

9. Because the type of cross-sectional study that is carried out by palaeoepidemiologists has no clear-cut end point, there is perhaps some justification in differentiating it from its modern counterpart and referring to it as a serrotic cross-sectional study. [For further details see T. Waldron, 'Prevalence Studies in Skeletal Populations: A Reply', *International Journal of Osteoarchaeology* 6 (1996): 320–32].

10. A more detailed index is the DMF calculated for each tooth surface, the DMFS. In this scheme, molars and pre-molars are considered to have five surfaces and the front teeth, four. The maximum value for DMFS for 28 teeth is 128. For further details see World Health Organisation, *Oral health surveys*, 3rd ed. (Geneva: WHO, 1987).

11. The DMF index is usually skewed to the right, and the presence of a substantial number of individuals with a very low index lowers the mean. To overcome this, a different measure has been suggested, the Significant Caries Index (SiC) which is the mean DMFT of the third of the study group with the highest caries score [D. Brathall,

'Introducing the Significant Caries Index Together with a Proposal for a New Global Oral Health Goal for 12-Year-Olds', *International Dental Journal* 50 (2000): 378–84]. Other measures have been proposed to take account of factors that give weights to decayed, filled, and sound teeth [see J. R. Jacobsen and R. J. Hunt, 'Validation of Oral Status Indicators', *Community Dental Health* 7 (1990): 279–84].

12. S. Hillson, *Dental Anthropology* (Cambridge: Cambridge University Press, 1996), pp. 280–84.

13. M. Tickle, K. Milson, D. King, P. Kearney-Mitchell, and A. Blinkhorn, 'The Fate of the Carious Teeth of Children Who Regularly Attend the General Dental Service', *British Dental Journal* 192 (2002): 219–23.

14. As a refinement, the DT can be calculated for molars, premolars and anterior teeth separately when the numerical value will be seen to fall from back to front.

15. There are some very elaborate systems for recording the site of caries on a tooth, and this is of particular interest to those studying the changes in the nature of caries over time. One of the most widely used is that published by W. J. Moor and M. E. Corbett ['Distribution of Dental Caries in Ancient British Populations: I. Anglo-Saxon Period', *Caries Research* 5 (1971): 151–68] but this is likely to be superseded by more recent schemes; see, for example, S. Hillson, 'Recording Dental Caries in Archaeological Human Remains', *International Journal of Osteoarchaeology* 11 (2001): 249–89.

16. The PMR is sometimes said to be 'denominator-free' because it does not require a knowledge of either the total population or the population at risk.

17. Until October 1992, the stillbirth rate included fetuses dying after the 28th week of pregnancy. Both the stillbirth and neonatal death rates were affected by this change, and not to everyone's delight [P. H. Cartlidge and J. H. Stewart, 'Effect of Changing the Stillbirth Definition on Evaluation of Perinatal Mortality Rates', *Lancet* 346 (1995): 486–88].

18. The current mean stillbirth rate in developing countries is approximately 12 per thousand, although there is a wide variation [J. Lawn, K. Shibuya, and C. Stein, 'No Cry at Birth: Global Estimates of Intrapartum Stillbirths and Intrapartum-Related Neonatal Deaths', *Bulletin of the World Health Organization* 83 (2005): 409–17; L. Say, A. Donner, A. Metin Gulmezoglu, M. Taljaard, and G. Piaggio, 'The Prevalence of Stillbirth: A Systematic Review', *Reproductive Health* 3 (2006); 1]. The stillbirth rate in England and Wales is currently 5.3 per thousand (*Childhood and Infant Deaths in 2001*, www.statistics.gov.uk/releases).

19. This is not *strictly* true; some cases arise as the result of trauma during adult life and some are secondary to degenerative changes in the spine. These varieties of spondylolysis, however, are by no means as numerous as the childhood cases, and we can safely ignore them for the sake of simplicity. See, for example, R. Cope, 'Acute Traumatic Spondylolysis: Report of a Case and Review of the Literature', *Clinical Orthopedics and Related Research* 230 (1988): 162–65; M. J. Herman and P. D. Pizzutillo, 'Spondylolysis and Spondylolisthesis in the Child and Adolescent: A New Classification, *Clinical Orthopedics and Related Research* 434 (2005): 46–54.

20. D. D'Ambrosia, 'Epidemiology of Osteoarthritis', *Orthopedics* 28 (2005): 2 Suppl., 205.

21. That is, unless they die as a result of their medication. For the minimal effects of osteoarthritis on survival see D. G. Manuel, W. Luo, A. M. Ugnat, and Y. Mao, 'Cause-Deleted Health-Adjusted Life Expectancy of Canadians with Selected Chronic Conditions', *Chronic Diseases in Canada* 24 (2003): 108–15.

22. This is a higher case-fatality rate that is reported in some of the clinical literature, but in many publications the rates are those that prevail in clinics where treatment is given and supervised; see, for example, D. Wilkinson and D. A. Moore, 'HIV-Related Tuberculosis in South Africa – Clinical Features and Outcome', *South African Medical Journal* 86 (1996): 64–7.

23. The data used here were abstracted from *Mortality and Causes of Death in South Africa, 1997 – 2003* (www.statssa.gov.za) and *Global Tuberculosis Control: Surveillance, Planning, Financing. WHO Report 2005* (Geneva: WHO, 2005).

24. Two relatively recent studies, one in a developed and the other in a developing country, suggest that about 2% of cases affect the skeleton [E. Pertuiset, J. Beaudreuil, F. Liote, et al., 'Spinal Tuberculosis in Adults: A Study of 103 Cases in a Developed Country, 1980 – 1994', *Medicine (Baltimore)* 78 (1999): 309–20; N. C. Mkandawire and E. Kaunda, 'Bone and Joint TB at Queen Elizabeth Central Hospital 1986 to 2002, *Tropical Doctor* 35 (2005): 14–16], whereas an older paper from Denmark, found that about 30% of cases did so [B. Autzen, J. J. Elberg, 'Bone and Joint Tuberculosis in Denmark', *Acta Paediatrica Scandinavica* 59 (1988): 50–2]. The lower estimate probably reflects earlier detection and better treatment but suggests that, in skeletal assemblages, the higher figure is more likely to obtain.

25. To obtain the correct denominators requires that the presence or absence of each joint is recorded; if information is required about the prevalence of disease within the separate compartments of a complex joint – the medial, lateral, and patello-femoral compartments of the knee, for example – these will have to be recorded separately. When reporting the prevalence in complex joints, one should report the combined prevalence of disease in *all* compartments; the prevalence in single compartments can be reported in addition, if there are valid reasons for doing so. What should *not* be done, since it can be very confusing and will prevent comparison with other studies, is to devise complicated scoring systems that amalgamate disease if it is present in more than one compartment. Thus, if one finds osteoarthritis to be present in both the medial and lateral compartments of the same knee, one can consider this *only* as a single case of osteoarthritis – not two – when expressing the prevalence of osteoarthritis of the knee. If authors depart from this practice, the reader may be left wondering what the rates really mean: see, for example, P. S. Bridges, 'Degenerative Joint Disease in Hunter-Gatherers and Agriculturalists from the Southeastern United States', *American Journal of Physical Anthropology* 85 (1991): 379–91.

26. In areas where tuberculosis is endemic, especially in the tropics, multiple lesions are more common than elsewhere, however [D. S. Chang, M. Rafii, G. McGuinness, and J. S. Jagirdar, 'Primary Multifocal Tuberculous Osteomyelitis with Involvement of the Ribs', *Skeletal Radiology* 27 (1998): 641–45].

27. A. Law, 'A Simple Method for Calculating the Prevalence of Disease in a Past Human Population', *International Journal of Osteoarchaeology* 15 (2005): 146–47; I assume the author's use of the term 'simple' in the title is ironic.

28. I am forgetting here those matters that were discussed in Chapter 2 and talking as though we have a representative sample of the potential whole assemblage. Those who wish to complicate things to an overwhelming degree can consider for themselves how they are going to deal with *those*; my guess is, that as good epidemiologists, they will ignore them and carry on regardless.

29. R. P. Davies, K. Torque, M. A. Bellis, T. Rimmington, and P. D. Davies, 'Historical Declines in Tuberculosis in England and Wales: Improving Social Conditions or

Natural Selection? *International Journal of Tuberculosis and Lung Disease* 3 (1999): 1051–54.

30. R. S. Guinto, J. A. Doull, and L. De Guia, 'Mortality of Persons with Leprosy Prior to Sulfone Therapy, Cordova and Talisay, Cebu, Philippines', *International Journal of Leprosy* 22 (1954): 273–84; K. H. Uttley, 'The Mortality from Leprosy in the Negro Populations of Antigua, West Indies, from 1857 to 1956', *Leprosy Review* 31 (1960): 193–99.

31. R. A. Kyle and E. D. Bayrd, 'Amyloidosis: Review of 236 Cases', *Medicine (Baltimore)* 54 (1975): 271–99.

Comparing Prevalences

One of the more interesting aspects of palaeoepidemiology is the comparison of frequency of disease within and between different groups to try to make inferences about the changing pattern of disease in the past and, perhaps, suggest possible causes for any observed fluctuations. To do this requires a high degree of comparability between studies with respect to both diagnosis and analysis.

A rough and ready way of comparing prevalence is to plot out, or simply examine, the 95% confidence intervals around a prevalence; if the confidence intervals overlap, then there is no statistically significant difference between them at the 5% level (that is to say $p > 0.05$). This is usually not a very satisfactory way of going about things, since the crude prevalence is almost always a poor summary statistic. Individual age- and sex-specific rates can be compared in this way, but this involves a great many comparisons, and there is some advantage in having a single summary rate to describe the experience of any entire assemblage that can then be used for comparative purposes.

The use of crude prevalence immediately presents a difficulty. For example, Table 5.1 shows the age-specific and crude prevalence for a disease in two hypothetical skeletal assemblages, A and B. The crude prevalence for A is 390.9 per thousand and for B, 343.0 per thousand, giving a rate ratio of 1.14 (with a 95% interval of 1.03 – 1.26) in favour of A.[1] In other words, it seems as though the disease is more common in A than in B. According to the age-specific prevalences in columns 3 and 6 of the table, however, this conclusion seems anomalous since, with the exception of the youngest group, they are actually lower in A than in B. Moreover, the age-structures of the two assemblages differ considerably, there being many

Table 5.1 Age-specific prevalences of disease in two populations

Age Group (years)	A			B		
	N (1)	n (2)	Rate/10³ (3)	N (4)	n (5)	Rate/10³ (6)
25–	32	2	62.5	49	3	61.2
35–	42	12	266.7	61	20	327.9
45–	58	27	465.5	30	16	533.3
55+	65	36	553.8	32	20	635.0
Total	197	77	390.9	172	59	343.0

N = total number in each age group
n = total number of cases
Rate ratio A:B = 1.14 (95% CI 1.03 – 1.26)

older individuals in A than in B and – conversely – many younger individuals in B than in A. And herein lies the basis of our problems: the disproportionate number of older individuals in A – in whom this particular disease is more common – is artificially elevating the crude prevalence. What is needed then, is some method that will make allowances for the different structures of the two groups and produce overall prevalences that are directly comparable. This is achieved either by some form of standardisation or by computing risk or odds ratios, methods that we discuss next.

Standardisation

There are two principal methods of standardisation, direct and indirect, and both need to be considered in some detail.

Direct Standardisation

In direct standardisation, the age-specific rates of the populations to be compared are applied in turn to a standard population to produce a standardised rate, sometimes called a comparative mortality figure. There are several potential choices for the standard population: it can be (1) entirely artificial; (2) a real population that may or may not be related to those under study; (3) one of the two groups actually being studied; or (4) both groups combined. For palaeoepidemiological purposes, the most convenient standard would be a combination of the two assemblages being compared.

The procedure to be used for direct standardisation can be illustrated using the population of the London Borough of Newham from the 2001 census. Column 2 of Table 5.2 shows the numbers in each of the four age groups at Newham corresponding to those for A and

Table 5.2 Directly standardised prevalences for populations A and B

Age Group (years)	N	n (rate A)	n (rate B)
25–	45765	2860.3	2800.8
35–	36731	9796.2	12044.1
45–	23787	11072.9	12685.6
55+	38024	20297.2	24145.2
Total	144307	44026.5	51675.8

N = total number in each age group in standard population (London Borough of Newham)
n (rate A) = number of cases obtained by applying age-specific prevalences from column 3 in Table 5.1
n (rate B) = number of cases obtained by applying age-specific prevalences from column 6 in Table 5.1
Standardised prevalence for A = 310.4 per thousand
Standardised prevalence for B = 358.1 per thousand
Standardised rate ratio = 0.87

B in Table 5.1. Columns 3 and 4 of Table 5.2 show the number of cases derived from multiplying column 2 by the age-specific rates for A and B (in columns 3 and 6 of Table 5.1). This yields a total of 44,027 cases using the rates for A, and 51,676 cases using the rates for B; thus there now appear to be more cases in B than in A. The standardised rate ratio (SRR) can be obtained by dividing the standardised overall prevalence for A by that for B:

$$\text{SRR} = \frac{310.4}{358.1} = 0.87$$

Thus, having made allowances for the different age-structures of A and B, we see that this particular disease is actually more common in B than in A, which is just what we would have expected from an examination of the age-specific rates in Table 5.1.[2]

One must keep in mind that standardised rates are artificial and do not imply anything about the true rates in the original populations, except their relationship to each other. Using a different standard population will yield different numbers of cases and different crude standardised rates, as can be seen from Table 5.3, where the standard is now the population of Christchurch, Hampshire, again from the 2001 census. The population of Christchurch is much smaller than that of Newham, so the number of cases obtained is smaller; the overall standardised rates for A and B are now 432 per thousand and 497 per thousand, respectively, but the standardised rate ratio is the same, 0.87.[3]

I said earlier that it is permissible to use one of the original populations, or both combined as the standard, and that this is the most convenient standard to use in palaeoepidemiology. Using A and B

Table 5.3 Directly standardised prevalences for populations A and B

Age Group (years)	N	n (rate A)	n (rate B)
25–	4355	266.5	266.5
35–	5540	1477.5	1816.6
45–	5580	2597.5	2975.8
55+	19146	10603.1	12157.7
Total	34612	14944.6	17216.6

N = total number in each age group in standard population (Christchurch, Hampshire)
n (rate A) = number of cases obtained by applying age-specific prevalences from column 3 in Table 5.1
n (rate B) = number of cases obtained by applying age-specific prevalences from column 6 in Table 5.1
Standardised prevalence for A = 431.9 per thousand
Standardised prevalence for B = 497.4 per thousand
Standardised rate ratio = 0.87

combined as the standard produces the results shown in Table 5.4; again, although the crude standardised rates are different, the SRR comes out once again as 0.87, showing that the arithmetic is correct. (For comparison, the crude prevalence and the various standardised rates are shown in Table 5.5.)

It should be clear from what has gone before that standardisation can be used only to compare two populations; if one wishes to compare the prevalence in more than two, then this has to be done in a pair-wise fashion comparing A with B, A with C, and B with C, for example. This can be rather cumbersome if several prevalences are to be compared, and the results are then usually best presented in the form of a matrix.

Table 5.4 Directly standardised prevalences for populations A and B

Age Group (years)	N	n (rate A)	n (rate B)
25–	81	5.1	5.0
35–	103	27.5	33.8
45–	88	41.0	46.9
55+	97	53.7	60.6
Total	369	127.3	146.3

N = total number in each age group in standard population (Populations A and B combined)
n (rate A) = number of cases obtained by applying age-specific prevalences from column 3 in Table 5.1
n (rate B) = number of cases obtained by applying age-specific prevalences from column 6 in Table 5.1
Standardised prevalence for A = 345.0 per thousand
Standardised prevalence for B = 396.5 per thousand
Standardised rate ratio = 0.87

Table 5.5 Summary of standardised prevalences for populations A and B with different standards[a]

Standard	Prevalence (per thousand)		SRR A:B
	A	B	
Original Populations	390.0	343.0	1.14
London Borough of Newham	310.4	358.1	0.87
Christchurch, Hampshire	431.9	497.4	0.87
A + B	345.0	396.5	0.87

[a]SRR = standardised rate ratio. The SRR comparing B:A is merely the reciprocal of 0.87 = 1.14.

It should also be clear that standardised rates cannot be compared between studies, unless the same standard has been used in each case. This is a problem that will seldom be encountered in palaeoepidemiology since standardised rates are almost never reported. If interstudy comparisons are to be made, however, a common standard should be agreed on and used, although it is hard to see that this would happen without an expert committee or two being convened. There seems little likelihood that this will happen any time soon, and for most purposes the combination of the two assemblages to be compared is the best – and most convenient – standard to use.

Indirect Standardisation

In a sense, indirect standardisation reverses the procedure followed in the direct method. The procedure for indirect standardisation is to apply age-specific rates from a standard population to each of the populations under study to produce what are referred to as *expected* numbers of cases, that is, the number of cases that would have occurred had the study population experienced the rates in the standard. The number of expected cases in each group is summed and compared with the number of cases actually observed to produce a standardised mortality (or morbidity) ratio, or SMR. The SMR[4] is simply derived as:

$$SMR = \frac{Observed}{Expected} \times 100$$

The procedure is illustrated in Table 5.6 with reference to our old friends A and B. In this instance, the age-specific rates of the standard population are shown in column 1 of the table and are applied in turn to each of the age groups to obtain the expected number of cases, shown in column 4 and 7; the observed numbers are given in

Table 5.6   Indirect standardisation of populations A and B

Age Group (years)	Standard Prevalence per Thousand (1)	A			B		
		N (2)	O (3)	E (4)	N (5)	O (6)	E (7)
25–	50.1	32	2	1.6	49	3	2.5
35–	375.6	42	12	15.8	61	20	22.9
45–	424.8	58	27	24.6	30	16	12.7
55+	591.4	65	36	38.4	32	20	18.9
Total			77	80.7		59	57.0

N = Total number in each age group (from Table 5.1)
O = number of cases observed (from Table 5.1)
E = number of cases expected by applying prevalences in column 1 to columns 2 and 5
SMR for A = 95.8
SMR for B = 103.5
Standardised rate ratio (SRR) = 0.92

the preceding columns. For A, the total expected number of cases is 80.7, and the total observed is 77; for B the numbers are 57 and 59, respectively. The SMR for A is thus 80.7/77 = 95.8, whereas for B, it is 59/57 = 103.5. The standardised rate ratio (SRR) is, therefore, 95.8/103.5 = 0.92 (95% CI 0.65 – 1.32).[5]

Note that, although indirect standardisation has a similar effect to the direct method in producing a standardised rate that is lower for A than for B, the rate ratio is different because neither the rates nor the populations to which they are applied are the same as in the direct method.

In modern epidemiology the indirect method is used much more frequently than the direct, particularly in occupational epidemiology, where the effects of exposure to harmful substances in the workplace are assessed.[6] Since the aim of these studies is most frequently to see how much an exposed population varies from normal, it is the age- and sex-specific rates of the disease under study in the general population that are used, although local rates may be used if they are available. What is often overlooked is that interstudy comparisons will be invalid unless the same rates are used in each study; it is not valid to compare SMRs directly, although this is very frequently done and reported in the literature where leagues tables of SMRs are compiled to show the supposed relative effects of a particular exposure on different populations.[7]

What is also often overlooked by those who use the indirect method it that the age-structure of the populations being compared affects the calculation of the expected numbers, and if it is markedly different, then an erroneous impression may be gained. I can illustrate this with the simple example shown in Table 5.7. Here we have two populations, C and D, with identical age-specific prevalences in the two subgroups, young and old, but with greatly different numbers in each group. The rates in the standard population (S), shown in column 3 of the table, are applied to each of the subgroups in turn to obtain the expected number of cases; these are 7.5 and 9 for C, and 45 and 15 for D. The SMRs are obtained as follows:

$$\text{SMR}_C = \frac{(9 + 150)}{(7.5 + 90)} = \frac{159}{97.5} \times 100 = 163.1$$

and

$$\text{SMR}_D = \frac{(54 + 25)}{(45 + 15)} = \frac{79}{60} \times 100 = 131.7$$

and the SRR = 1.24.

These results suggest that the disease is more common in C than in D, which is obviously not the case since the age-specific rates are the same in both. The anomaly results from the difference in the disparity in the numbers in the age groups. If the rates are standardised directly to population S, the standardised rate for both C and D is 37.3 per thousand, and the SRR is – of course – unity, which is what the age-specific rates would have led us to believe in the first instance.

The lesson is that SMRs cannot be directly compared unless the age-structure of the populations being compared is similar, or unless age-specific SMRs are compared; this is a rather cumbersome procedure, however, and most investigators would prefer to work with a summary measure.

Table 5.7 Indirect standardisation of two populations

	Standard (S)			C			D		
Age Group	N	n	P	N	n	P	N	n	P
Young	2000	30	15	500	9	18	3000	54	18
Old	6000	180	30	3000	150	50	500	25	50
Total	8000	210	23.3	3500	159	45.4	3500	79	22.6

N = total number in each age group
n = number of cases in each age group
P = prevalence per thousand
SMR for C = 163.1
SMR for D = 131.7
Standardised rate ratio = 1.24
By *direct* standardisation on population S, the overall standardised prevalence for both C and D = 37.3 and the SRR = unity.

Table 5.8 Indirect standardisation using combined prevalences of A and B

Age Group (years)	Prevalence per Thousand for A + B	A		B	
		O	E	O	E
25–	61.7	2	2.0	3	3.0
35–	213.6	12	9.0	20	13.0
45–	488.6	27	28.3	16	14.7
55+	577.3	36	37.5	20	18.5
Total		77	76.8	59	49.2

O = number of cases observed
E = number of cases expected using combined prevalence
SMR for A = 1003
SMR for B = 119.9
Standardised rate ratio (SRR) = 0.84

A problem of particular relevance to palaeoepidemiologists is the choice of rates to use for indirect standardisation. In any kind of morbidity study it is often difficult to find access to population morbidity data, and certainly none exists for assemblages of human remains. The most straightforward solution is to use the combined age-specific prevalences of the two populations. This has been done for populations A and B in Table 5.8, which shows the combined rates and the observed and expected numbers. The SMR for A now becomes 100.3 and for B, 119.9. These are different from those computed earlier, and the SRR is now 0.84 (95% CI 0.59 – 1.19).

Risk and Odds Ratios

Prevalences can also be compared using risk or odds ratios. For example, suppose that we have two populations with age-specific prevalences $p_1 \ldots p_i$ and $q_1 \ldots q_i$. To compare the prevalences we could calculate the risk ratios:

$$\frac{p_1}{q_1} \ldots \frac{p_1}{q_i}$$

or the odds ratios:

$$\frac{p_1/(1 - p_1)}{q_1/(1 - q_1)} \ldots \frac{p_i/(1 - p_i)}{q_i/(1 - q_i)}$$

Generally, calculation of the odds ratio (OR) is to be preferred, because the age-specific prevalences of many of the common diseases encountered in human remains are likely to vary considerably.[8] The odds ratio for each age-stratum can be summed to give a common odds ratio that combines the age-specific prevalences in two populations into a single summary statistic.[9]

From Table 5.1 the age-specific odds ratios can be derived as follows. For those aged 25 – 34 the ratio is

$$\frac{62.5/(1000 - 62.5)}{61.2/(1000 - 61.2)} = 1.03$$

For the succeeding age-strata, the odds ratios are as follows: for ages 35 – 44, 0.75; for ages 45 – 54, 0.76; and for ages 55+, 0.74.

The common odds ratio is obtained by summing the individual rates thus:

$$\left(\frac{62.5/937.5}{61.2/938.8}\right) + \left(\frac{266.7/733.3}{327.9/672.1}\right) + \left(\frac{465.5/534.5}{533.3/466.7}\right) + \left(\frac{533.8/466.2}{625.0/375.0}\right)$$

This can be rearranged to:

$$\frac{(62.5 \times 938.8) + (266.7 \times 672.1) + (465.5 \times 466.7) + (533.8 \times 375.0)}{(61.2 \times 937.5) + (327.9 \times 733.3) + (534.5 \times 533.3) + (466.2 \times 625.0)}$$

and, finally:

$$\text{Common Odds Ratio} = \frac{655\,348}{874\,248} = 0.75$$

The 95% confidence interval can be calculated for the common odds ratio, and, in the case above, the limits are 0.68 – 0.83.

From this result it can be seen that the prevalence in A is actually substantially lower than in B, and, since the confidence interval does not include unity, the difference is statistically significant at the 5% level.

The odds ratio can, of course, be calculated in the inverse sense that it has been done here, that is, with the rates for B as the numerators and those for A as the denominators. Rather than do the sums all over again, it is simplest to take the reciprocal of the common odds ratio shown above, which is then 1.33, confirming again that the rates are higher in B than in A.

Which Method of Comparison to Use?

The odds ratio method is probably the best one to use to compare prevalence in two assemblages. The common odds ratio provides a simple summary statistic with a 95% confidence interval, which expresses the difference between two groups and is easy to understand. Where three (or more) groups are to be compared, a common odds ratio can be calculated for the first and second, first and third, and so on, and the results can be presented in the form of a matrix.

The indirect method of standardisation was for many years the method preferred by modern epidemiologists, but it has come in for a lot of criticism. As long ago as 1923 Wolfenden wrote that 'it should be substituted for the direct method... only after due examination', and Yule noted in 1934 that it was safe 'only for the comparison of single pairs of populations'.[10] Not daunted by these warnings, epidemiologists, and especially occupational epidemiologists, continued to use SMRs fearlessly and often incorrectly, ignoring further strictures by more recent authorities such as Rothman, who declared that 'a common standard should be employed, and comparison of SMRs should be avoided'.[11] On balance, there is not much to commend the indirect method in palaeoepidemiology; if the common odds ratio is not used, then the direct form of standardisation is the next best option.

If a form of standardisation is used, there will be some difficulty in finding prevalences for the diseases that are likely to be of interest to palaeoepidemiologists, and, to my knowledge, there has been none published for skeletal assemblages that could be used as standard rates. In both forms of standardisation, the easiest option for the investigator is to use either the combined groups or the combined age-specific prevalences as the standards, recognising that this would preclude direct comparison with other studies.

With direct standardisation it is possible to take any population, real or imaginary, as the standard, and if this could become the agreed reference datum, so that all investigators used it, then direct interstudy comparisons would be possible. Given how difficult it is for those who study human remains to agree about almost anything, the chances that such a suggestion would meet universal support is vanishingly small.

A Few Cautionary Notes

One drawback to the direct method of standardisation that has not been mentioned so far is that when the number of individuals in a subgroup is very small, the prevalence can appear to be remarkably high if only a few cases are present. Where it seems likely that a high prevalence is the result of the small numbers in one or more subgroups of one of the study groups, it would be prudent either to wait until the number can be enhanced by the examination of more skeletons or to combine age groups to swell the numbers.

Whether the common odds ratio or direct standardisation is used to compare prevalences, there is one further disadvantage that should be mentioned, which relates to a potential loss of information. For example, it may be the case that a disease is equally prevalent in the younger age groups of two assemblages but substantially different in the older individuals. Although this difference will be reflected in both the common odds ratio and the SRR, there will be no information as to where the difference arises. In another case, a disease may be substantially more common in the young individuals of one group than another but much less common in the elderly. The common odds ratio or the SRR may thus be close to unity, totally obscuring some extremely interesting difference. On this account it may be best always to compare age-specific odds ratios as well as the common odds ratio, proving that the size of the different age classes is sufficient to provide a reliable estimate, and provided that you have an indulgent editor.

Endnotes

1. It is perfectly permissible, of course, to rearrange the rate ratio to illustrate that the disease is *less* common in B; if this is done, the rate ratio is 0.88 (the reciprocal of the ratio of 1.14 reported in the text).

2. The 95% confidence interval can – of course – be calculated; in this case it is 0.77 – 0.97. The significance between rates can be determined using Cochrane's test; see P. Armitage and G. Berry, *Statistical Methods in Medical Research*, 2nd ed. (Oxford: Blackwell, 1987). A more mathematical treatment of standardisation is to be found in Rothman and Greenland, *Ibid.*, especially Chapters 3 and 4.

3. These two populations were chosen because whereas the population of Newham is heavily weighted toward the young, that of Christchurch has an abundance of the elderly. The data were downloaded from www.statistics.gov.uk/census2001.

4. Although it is usual for the division sum to be multiplied by 100, there are occasions in the literature where this is not done.

5. The fact that the 95% confidence interval contains 1 indicates that the difference between the two hypothetical rates is not statistically significant; scarcely surprising when one considers how close they are. To test if an individual SMR differs significantly from 100, a chi-squared test can be used with 1 degree of freedom, where $\chi^2 = $ (Observed-Expected)^2/Expected. In the case of A, $\chi^2 = (77 – 80.7)^2/80.7 = 13.7/80.7 = 0.17$. This hypothetical rate is obviously not significantly different from 100. (With 1 degree of freedom any chi-squared result less than 3.84 is not significant at the 5% level.)

6. For examples of occupational epidemiology see H. Checkoway, N. Pearce, and D. Kriebel, *Research Methods in Occupational Epidemiology* (Oxford: Oxford Univeristy Press, 2004) and R. R. Monson, *Occupational Epidemiology* (Boca Raton, FL: CRC Press, 1990).

7. In the first edition of *Modern Epidemiology* (published in 1986), which Rothman wrote on his own, he had very strong words to say about the habit of his colleagues in comparing SMRs. In the second edition, which is a multiauthored volume, and much the worse for it, this stricture no longer seems to appear, perhaps because he mellowed in the 12 years between editions, or more likely he gave up because it hurt too much to keep knocking his head against the brick wall.

8. For further discussion of risk and odds ratios see H. A. Kahn and C. T. Sempos, *Statistical Methods in Epidemiology* (New York: Oxford University Press, 1989).

9. The calculation of the common odds ratio is derived from N. Mantel and W. Haenszel, 'Statistical Aspects of the Analysis of Data from Retrospective Studies of Disease', *Journal of the National Cancer Institute* 22 (1959): 719–48. Further details of this method of comparing prevalences can be found in D. Clayton and M. Hills, *Statistical Methods in Epidemiology* (Oxford: Oxford University Press, 1993).

10. H. H. Wolfenden, 'On the Methods of Comparing the Mortalities of Two or More Communities, and the Standardization of Death Rates', *Journal of the Royal Statistical Society* 86 (1923): 399–411; G. Yule, 'On Some Points Relating to Vital Statistics, More Especially Statistics of Occupational Mortality', *Journal of the Royal Statistical Society* 97 (1934): 1–84.

11. This is to be found in the first edition of Rothman, *Modern Epidemiology*, (1986), p. 49.

6 | Proportional Mortality and Morbidity

When comparing the frequency of disease between populations, use the population size in the denominator. However, occasional uncertainties arise about the denominator, and this may be particularly the case with skeletal assemblages. Under these circumstances it is permissible to compare the proportional mortality or morbidity. The proportional mortality is simply the proportion of all deaths attributed to a particular cause within a population;[1] that is to say

$$PM = \frac{\text{Number of deaths attributed to a specific cause}}{\text{Total number of deaths}} \times 100$$

where PM = proportional mortality. Note that the calculation of PM takes no account of the size of the population in which the deaths occurred, and so it is often referred to as a denominator-free statistic.

Some hypothetical proportional mortality data are shown in Table 6.1 for two populations, E and F. It can be seen that, although heart disease accounts for the greatest proportion of deaths in both populations, the rank order for the remaining causes is considerably different; most notably deaths from trauma seem to be much less frequent in F and in E. The proportions of trauma in the two populations can readily be compared by calculating the proportional mortality ratio (PMR). In this case,

$$PMR = \frac{\text{Proportion of trauma in E}}{\text{Proportion of trauma in F}} = \frac{27}{5} \times 100 = 540$$

Table 6.1 Specific causes of death as a proportion of all causes for two populations

| | E | | | F | | |
Cause of Death	Number of Deaths	Proportion of Total Deaths	Rank Order	Number of Deaths	Proportion of Total Deaths	Rank Order
Cancer	27,000	18	3	35,100	27	2
Heart disease	48,000	32	1	62,400	48	1
Respiratory disease	13,500	9	4=	3,900	3	6
Hepatic disease	7,500	5	6	7,800	6	4
Trauma	40,500	27	2	6,500	5	5
All other causes	13,500	9	4=	14,300	11	3
	150,000	100		130,000	100	

This is the simplest case, but it is also possible to calculate the PMR by deriving an expected number of deaths and comparing it with those observed. Returning to the data in Table 6.1, we see that if the rate of trauma in F were applied to E, then the number of trauma cases expected would be 7,500. In fact, the number observed was 40,500, so that if

$$PMR = \frac{Observed}{Expected} \times 100$$

then

$$PMR = \frac{40,500}{7,500} = 540 \ (95\% \ CI \ 535 - 545)$$

The PMR is the same as given earlier, as would be expected. The advantage of using this method is that age- and sex-specific expected numbers can be generated when the expected number overall will simply be the sum of the expected numbers obtained for each age- and sex-specific stratum.

It will not have escaped the reader's notice that the PMR obtained this way is similar to the method used for calculating the SMR; Decoufle and his colleagues[2] have shown that there is a relationship between the PMR and the SMR such that

$$PMR = \frac{1}{k}SMR$$

where k is a constant that is approximately equivalent to the age-adjusted overall SMR. Where $k = 1$, then the PMR and the SMR are equal.

Mortality Odds Ratio

In 1981, Miettinen and Wang[3] introduced what they called the mortality odds ratio (MOR) as an alternative to the PMR, about which they expressed a number of reservations. Firstly they argued that the PMR was not a quality with any intrinsic interest, being used only as a surrogate for the SMR, which they considered to be a more useful and informative measure. Secondly they were dismissive of the PMR on the grounds that it is dependent on how common other causes of death are, relative to the disease of interest. They proposed instead that the mortality odds ratio should be used, since this would be analogous to the odds ratio in a case-control study.

The calculation is the same as for the odds ratio in a case-control study (see Chapter 7). The number of cases whose cause of death is the object of the study is determined in each of two groups (exposed and non-exposed in an occupational study, for example), and the number of all other causes of death is also established. As we see in Table 6.1 again, the MOR for traumatic deaths is

$$\frac{40,500/109,500}{6,500/123,500}$$

which simplifies to

$$\frac{40,500 \times 123,500}{6,500 \times 109,500} = 7.03 \,(95\% \text{ CI } 6.84 - 7.22)$$

Limitations of the Use of the PMR

There are a number of limitations in the use of the PMR. Firstly, it is valid only if the deaths rates in the two populations being compared are similar. Secondly, since the proportions of deaths must necessarily add up to 100, any increase in the proportions of deaths from one cause must be accompanied by a decrease in the proportion of deaths from other causes. From a simple examination of the data it will not always be clear whether an increased proportion is real or apparent; clarity can be achieved only if the cause-specific death rates are known, and it is usually because they are *not* known that the PMR is used in the first case. It is also important in a proportional mortality study that the causes of death are diagnosed and classified in the same way in the populations being compared; to do otherwise – of course – deprives the results of the comparison of any value.

In palaeoepidemiology it is not possible to carry out mortality studies, but it is reasonable under some circumstances to carry out proportional morbidity studies and calculate a *morbidity* odds ratio to compare the frequency of two conditions. For example, consider the occurrence of spondylolysis in two assemblages. In the first there are 10 cases and 466 other conditions; in the second there are 13 cases and 231 other types of pathology.[4] The MOR is 0.38 (95% CI 0.17 – 0.88) suggesting that spondylolysis is significantly less frequent in the first than in the second assemblage.[5]

Calculating the MOR seems about as simple and straightforward a procedure as can be imagined, but some thought has to be given to deciding exactly what constitutes a 'disease' or a 'condition'. There is very little difficulty with examples of gross pathology, but with many conditions there is no dichotomous state of 'present' or 'absent'; do minute osteophytes or a tiny trace of periosteal new bone count as a disease or not? And is one counting *all* different conditions, in which case the number of conditions is likely to be several times greater than the number of skeletons in the assemblage, or simply the number of diseased skeletons? I think that the reader should by now know the answer to that question.

In practice, the differentiation between normal and abnormal tends to be somewhat arbitrary and differs from one observer to another. So long as the strategy for distinguishing between normal and abnormal is codified before the start of the study (preferably by using operational definitions), a disease will be defined by the rules laid down and the analysis will be valid – so long as the rules are adhered to. When more than one observer is involved in the study, interobserver error tests must be carried out before the main study is started, and any differences between observers must be clarified.

Missing data can cause problems, but only if the preservation of the two groups differs substantially. If it does not, then it is probably permissible to make the assumption that any loss of information will tend to cancel out and there will be no bias in the study on this account. This requires some preliminary assessment of the material; if it is found that there is a marked disparity between the assemblages, this would suggest that one would be more fruitfully employed doing something else.

Ranking

Another way of examining data without using denominators is by means of ranking. For example, suppose that the frequencies with which various joints were affected by osteoarthritis (OA) in a group of medieval assemblages were ranked as shown in Table 6.2. A group of postmedieval assemblages is then examined and the rank order of the joints affected in these remains compared with the medieval assemblages; see column 3 of Table 6.2. There are certainly some differences in ranking; thus OA of the hip is ranked fourth in the medieval assemblages but only eighth in the postmedieval; conversely, OA of the foot slips up the rankings (from eight to fourth) in the postmedieval period. A number of other changes in ranking can be noted, but what we would like to know is whether or not these changes are due to chance or whether there is a significant difference that might indicate a change in the expression of the disease. There are a number of ways in which the rankings can be examined

Table 6.2 Rank order of joints affected by osteoarthritis in medieval and post-medieval skeletal assemblages

Rank Order	Medieval	Postmedieval	D	D^2
1	Shoulder	Shoulder	0	0
2	Spine	Spine	0	0
3	Hand	Hand	0	0
4	Hip	Foot	−4	16
5	Knee	SCJ	−1	1
6	SCJ	Knee	+1	1
7	Wrist	TMJ	−3	9
8	Foot	Hip	+4	16
9	Elbow	Elbow	0	0
10	TMJ	Wrist	+3	9

SCJ = sterno-clavicular joint
TMJ = temporo-mandibular joint
D = difference in rank
D^2 = difference in rank squared

statistically.[6] The sign test can be used, but probably the simplest method is to calculate Spearman's rank correlation coefficient (r_s). To do this, note the differences in rank for each of the joints affected (D) and square the difference (D^2) (see Table 6.2). Spearman's coefficient is then calculated as:

$$r_s = 1 - \frac{6 \sum D^2}{N(N^2 - 1)}$$

where N = number of ranks. For the example in Table 6.2

$$r_s = 1 - \frac{6 \times 52}{10(99)} = 1 - \frac{312}{990} = 1 - 0.32 = 0.68.$$

This value of r_s indicates that the two rankings are highly positively correlated and the correlation coefficient is statistically significant ($p < 0.05$) indicating that the differences seen are most likely due to chance.

Endnotes

1. In the case of proportional morbidity, the number of cases of a particular disease forms the numerator and the total number of all diseases the denominator.

2. P. Decoufle, T. L. Thomas, and L. W. Pickle, 'Comparison of the Proportional Mortality Ratio and Standardized Mortality Ratio Risk Measures', *American Journal of*

Epidemiology 111 (1980): 263–69; O. Wong and P. Decoufle, 'Methodological Issues Involving the Standardized Mortality Ratio and Proportionate Mortality Ratio in Occupational Studies', *Journal of Occupational Medicine* 24 (1982): 299–304.

3. O. S. Miettenen and J.-D. Wang, 'An Alternative to the Proportionate Mortality Ratio', *American Journal of Epidemiology* 114 (1981): 144–48.

4. These data are from an actual study that was published some years ago [T. Waldron, 'Variations in the Rates of Spondylolysis in Early Populations', *International Journal of Osteoarchaeology* 1 (1991): 63–65].

5. Conversely of course, one could argue that the condition was significantly *higher* in the second population than in the first. The MOR in this case is the reciprocal of 0.38, that is, 2.62 (95% CI 1.13 – 6.07). The way in which the odds ratio is calculated depends on the hypothesis under test.

6. S. Siegel and N. J. Castellan, *Nonparametric Statistics for the Behavioral Sciences*, 2nd ed. (New York: McGraw Hill, 1988), Chapter 9.

Analytical Epidemiology

A distinction is sometimes made between descriptive methods in epidemiology, such as the determination of incidence and prevalence, and analytical methods in which hypotheses are said to be tested. Although there is very little to be said to justify this distinction, it has become enshrined in epidemiological folklore, and I have bowed to the convention by discussing the concept under this head. In most analytical studies, the hypothesis to be tested relates to the aetiology of a particular disease, or a group of diseases – the cause of specific cancers, or relationships between certain dietary items and heart disease, for example.

There is a somewhat limited opportunity to use analytical methods in palaeoepidemiology, but this is probably all the more reason for using such opportunities as we do have, and I will illustrate some in what follows. The type of study that is used is referred to as a case-control, or case-referent study, and much of this chapter describes this particular entity;[1] we will also touch on the differences between the odds ratio and the risk ratio.

The Case-Control Study

The case-control study has several attractions for the epidemiologist. It is relatively cheap, it can be conducted much more quickly than a follow-up study as a rule, and it is particularly useful for investigating rare diseases. The way in which a case-control study is undertaken is conceptually the reverse of the cohort study. In the latter, one begins by defining an exposure and then goes on to follow up a cohort with this exposure to measure the outcome variable of interest. In a case-control study, the starting point is the outcome, and then one seeks retrospectively to determine the exposure that produced it, using exposure in a very broad sense (Figure 7.1). The advantage in the case-control approach can readily be seen by considering a rare disease such as leukaemia. There are rather less than 4,000 cases of leukaemia newly diagnosed in the United Kingdom each year, about a third of which are acute myeloid leukaemia.[2] There is some suggestion that exposure to organic solvents may increase the risk of developing acute myeloid leukaemia; with about 2.5 million workers

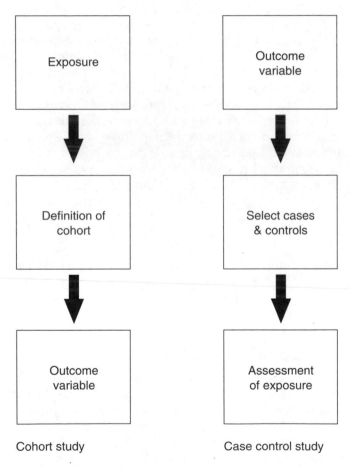

Figure 7.1 Diagrammatic representation of a cohort study and a case-control study

in the United Kingdom exposed to solvents, some 250 cases would arise annually, given that the incidence is approximately 100 per million. Even with a two-fold increase in risk, to be sure of detecting 100 cases a year would involve following up 500,000 workers exposed to solvents, a task that would stagger the imagination of investigator and funding body alike. Much simpler to start at the other end, and collect cases of leukaemia and determine the proportion with significant solvent exposure.[3]

The cohort study starts with defining an exposure and following up an exposed cohort to determine the number developing the outcome variable of interest. The case-control study starts by defining those with the outcome variable of interest, matching with controls and determining exposure in both cases and controls.

The study group in a case-control study are cases that have been selected as fulfilling certain entry criteria that have been determined at the start of the study. The cases may be either incident or prevalent, incident cases being those newly arising and prevalent cases those already diagnosed. The majority of case-control studies use prevalent cases, and invariably do so when the disease is rare.[4] It should be obvious that the entry criteria must be strictly adhered to, but it is surprising how often they are relaxed when it becomes difficult to recruit a sufficient number of cases into the study.

Having recruited the cases, the controls are selected so that they match the cases in as many ways as possible, except of course that they do *not* have the disease under study. Surprisingly, the selection of the controls may present considerable difficulty, and it is by no means always clear how they should be drawn. Matching on age and sex are usually obvious criteria to use, but the closer the matching, the less likely there is to be any difference between the cases and the controls with the potential for the loss of interesting or important information. For example, matching on smoking habits in a study of tumours might obscure the contribution made by smoking to the aetiology of the disease; the problems of this so-called over-matching are discussed in epidemiological texts to which reference should be made for further details.[5] The criteria by which controls are selected in many modern studies are very much more relaxed than was formerly the case.

Once the cases and controls have been selected, the investigator moves on to the next stage of the study, which is to determine what events or exposures each might have experienced. This is achieved most often through the use of a questionnaire that is given to both cases and controls, preferably by a member of the investigating team who is blind as to the status of the individual being questioned; this is to avoid observer bias as far as possible. Increasingly, use is also now being made of genetic or other biomarkers to study, for example, the aetiology of cancer,[6] infections,[7] and the risks from environmental or occupational exposures.[8] This is the relatively new variant known as molecular epidemiology, which is certain to have much wider application in the future.

The nature of the information to be collected from the study-base depends on the aim of the study, and investigators sometimes differentiate between hypothesis-generating studies and hypothesis-testing studies. An hypothesis-generating study might be established because a view has been formed that – let's say – asthma is related to working in a particular industry. Cases of asthma will be selected with their controls, and the numbers working in that industry will be determined. But the questionnaire will include not only the bald question, do you or have you ever worked in industry A, but a great many other questions about work, exposures at work, personal habits, hobbies, and so on. A great number of variables will be entered into the analysis, from which one hopes that more specific clues will arise. It may be found, for example, that only those who undertake a particular job in the industry are really at risk. Having found this, the investigators will then almost certainly wish to go on to carry out an hypothesis-testing study in which they concentrate on the particular risk they have found previously. And to do this they should recruit any entirely new study-base; subjects used in an hypothesis-generating study are excluded from the hypothesis-testing study.

Questionnaires, which should have been validated before the study starts, may be administered directly, over the telephone, or by post, the cost diminishing from first to last. The best information will be obtained from a directly administered questionnaire, and, certainly when self-administered, the accuracy and completeness of the answers will be inversely related to the length and complexity of the form. When more than one investigator is involved in collecting information, they must be properly trained to ensure that their results are as free from bias as possible. Molecular epidemiology requires that biological samples of some kind are taken, and these should be dealt with in the same laboratory, using the same protocol for all samples.

At some point, the investigator will have obtained information on the numbers of cases and controls who fall into each of the exposure groups; so many will have been exposed to aluminium dust, or taken a particular drug, or have had measles, and so on. The trick now is to

Table 7.1 Number of cases and controls with exposure to coal dust

	Exposure	No Exposure	Total
Cases	27	173	200
Controls	11	189	200
Total	38	362	400

$\chi^2 = 7.43, p < 0.01$
Odds ratio = 2.68 (95% CI 1.29 – 5.57)

see whether there are differences in the number of cases exposed, compared with the controls, and, if so, whether this difference matters; this last factor is usually expressed in terms of statistical significance. The simplest way of testing this is with the chi-squared (χ^2) statistic. Suppose that in a study of exposure to coal dust and asthma, there were 200 cases and 200 controls and that 27 of the cases had exposure to coal dust, whereas this was so for only 11 of the controls. The results come down to a simple 2 x 2 table (Table 7.1), and χ^2 with 1 degree of freedom is 7.43, a highly significant result ($p < 0.01$), indicating that the exposure is very likely to be causally related to the development of asthma. A result of this significance would certainly lead the investigator to declare that coal dust *did* cause asthma and form the basis of his next – much larger – grant application.[9]

Confounding

One of the issues that must be considered in a case-control study is that of confounding. A confounding factor – or confounder – is one that satisfies two conditions: (1) it is a risk factor for the disease under study and (2) it is associated with the study exposure but is not a consequence of it. In practice, it has become more usual to apply a more restricted definition of a confounder as one that produces the same outcome as the exposure under study. This is actually a definition of an effect-modifier, but the confusion is now so widespread and so commonly applied, that there is no going back from it.[10] One common confounder in modern epidemiological studies is smoking. In a study of lung cancer, for example, smoking habits would have a potentially confounding effect on the outcome and cases, and either controls would have to be matched for smoking habits or smoking would have to be allowed for in the statistical analysis. There are a number of ways in which this can be done, but the most common procedure and one that would suit almost all palaeoepidemiological applications is the Mantel-Haenszel chi-squared test.[11]

Table 7.2 Number of cases and controls with exposure to coal dust and birds

	Coal Dust Exposure	No Coal Dust Exposure	Total
Cases			
Bird fancier	11	18	29
Not bird fancier	16	155	171
Controls			
Bird fancier	0	5	5
Not bird fancier	11	184	195
Total	38	362	400

$\chi^2 = 3.47$ ($p > 0.05$)
Odds ratio = 2.07 (95% CI = 0.96 – 4.48)

To see the Mantel-Haenszel (M-H) test in action, suppose that from our study of asthma and exposure to coal dust we reanalysed the data and found that a substantial number of individuals were pigeon fanciers; it is not at all unreasonable to assume that keeping pigeons would result in exposure to bird proteins and that this might provoke an immune response giving rise to the development of asthma. The data could be stratified to take account of this possible confounding factor (Table 7.2). Of the cases, 27 have had exposure to coal dust, whereas 29 were bird fanciers. For the controls, the corresponding figures are 11 and 5, respectively. Using the M-H procedure, $\chi^2 = 3.47$, which is a nonstatistically significant result. In other words, having allowed for the exposure to bird proteins, there is no significant difference between the cases and controls with respect to their coal dust exposure.[112]

The Odds Ratio

As well as analysing the results of a case-control study with the M-H χ^2, the odds ratio can also be calculated. The odds ratio is the ratio of the probability that an event will occur to the probability that it will not. The odds ratio (OR) is often confused with the relative risk, or risk ratio (RR), and some authors tend to use the terms synonymously. The differences between the two can be illustrated by reference to Table 7.3. In this table, the odds of cases being exposed is a/c, and the odds of the controls being exposed is b/d. The odds ratio then, is

$$\frac{a/c}{b/d} = \frac{ad}{bc}$$

Table 7.3 Relationship between odds ratio and relative risk

		Outcome		
		+	−	
Exposure	+	a	b	$a+b$
	−	c	d	$c+d$
		$a+c$	$c+d$	$a+b+c+d$

Odds ratio $= \dfrac{a/c}{b/d} = \dfrac{ad}{bc}$

Relative risk $= \dfrac{a/(a+b)}{c/(c+d)}$

The risk of developing the outcome in the exposed group is $a/(a+b)$, and in the non-exposed group, the risk is $c/(c+d)$. The relative risk, therefore, is

$$\frac{a/(a+b)}{c/(c+d)}$$

The formulae for calculating the two estimates are different, but under the very rare condition in which a and c are very small compared with b and d, then

$$a + b \approx a$$

and

$$c + d \approx d$$

The relative risk then becomes $(a/b)/(c/d)$ or, ad/bc, which is identical to the formula for the odds ratio. Thus, given a rare condition the odds ratio approximates to the relative risk, and hence the basis for the interchangeable use of the two terms should be restricted to these circumstances only.

Referring back to Tables 7.1 and 7.2, we see that the odds ratio in the first case is 2.68 (95% CI 1.29 – 5 57), whereas in the second the odds ratio is 2.07 (95% CI 0.96 – 4.48). Since the first confidence interval does not include unity, its associated odds ratio would be considered statistically significant (at the 5% level); however, since the second confidence interval does contain unity, this odds ratio is not significant.

Differences between the Relative Risk and the Odds Ratio

Putting some data into a table demonstrates some other differences between the relative risk and the odds ratio. Consider the case in which the relationship between asthma and hay fever has been

Table 7.4 Association between hay fever and asthma in a study population

		Asthma +	Asthma –	Total
Hay fever	+	25	347	372
	–	90	788	878
	Total	115	1,135	1,250

Odds ratio of an individual with hay fever having asthma = 0.63
Relative risk of an individual with hay fever having asthma = 0.66
Odds ratio of an individual with asthma having hay fever = 0.63
Relative risk of an individual with asthma having hay fever = 0.71

studied, with the results set out in Table 7.4. From this table we see that the probability that an individual with hay fever will also have asthma is 25/372; the probability of an individual without hay fever having asthma is 90/878. The relative risk is thus (25/372)/(90/878) = 0.66. The odds ratio is (25/347)/(90/788) = (25 × 788)/(90 × 347) = 0.63. If we look at the table the other way round, what is the probability of an individual with asthma having hay fever? This time it is 25/115, and the probability of an individual without asthma having hay fever is 347/1135. The relative risk is now (25/115)/(347/1135) = 0.71. The odds ratio is (25/90)/(347/788) = (25 × 788)/(90 × 347) = 0.63. Therefore, whichever way one looks at the table, the OR is the same, but the RR is different.[13]

The Case-Control Study in Palaeoepidemiology

As I mentioned at the start of this chapter, the use of the case-control study is rather restricted in palaeoepidemiology by the nature of the material with which we have to deal, but that ought only to encourage the use of the method where it *can* be helpful. In palaeoepidemiology the case-control approach can be used *inter alia* to test associations between conditions or to test the proposition that a disease may be more common in one group than another.

There are almost no examples of case-control studies applied to skeletal assemblages, but I can illustrate the first type of example mentioned above with a study of my own and supply some hypothetical data to illustrate the second.

In the clinical literature there are several instances in which spondylolysis or spondylolisthesis has been found in association with spina bifida occulta; the proportion of those with spondylolysis in whom spina bifida also occurs has been quoted to be in the range of 13 – 70%. There is also some evidence that the prevalence of transitional vertebrae is lower in patients with spondylolysis than in controls. These lesions are all readily identified in the skeleton, and since none is all that common, a case-control approach is well suited to study the reported associations.[14]

To be included in the study, skeletons with spondylolysis (the cases) were required to have an intact sacrum so that presence or absence of spina bifida and transitional vertebrae could be established. Sixty-four cases were found from different archaeological sites. All were adult and for each case, two controls were randomly chosen from among the remaining adult skeletons at the appropriate site; no matching was undertaken, but allowances for any sex differences were made in the analysis.

The results of the study are shown in Tables 7.5 and 7.6, stratified for sex. Among the cases, 43 were male and 21 female; the corresponding numbers among the controls were 79 and 49, respectively. Five of the cases had spina bifida as did 9 of the controls; the OR was 1.10 with a 95% CI of 0.30 – 3.90. Only 2 of the cases had transitional vertebrae, compared with 11 of the controls. In this case the OR was 0.32 (95% CI 0.07 – 1.50), another nonsignificant result. This

Table 7.5 Number of cases and controls with spina bifida

		Spina Bifida	
		+	−
Cases	Male	4	39
	Female	1	20
Controls	Male	6	73
	Female	3	46

Odds ratio = 1.10, 95%; CI = 0.35 – 3.44

Table 7.6 Number of cases and controls with transitional vertebrae

		Transitional Vertebrae	
		+	−
Cases	Male	2	41
	Female	0	21
Controls	Male	9	70
	Female	2	47

Odds ratio = 0.32, 95% CI = 0.07 – 1.50

Table 7.7 Results of a case-control study of diffuse idiopathic skeletal hyperostosis (DISH) and social status

	Religious/High Status	Low Status	Total
Case	18	25	43
Control	7	79	86
Total	25	104	129

$\chi^2 = 20.70$, $p < 000.1$.
Odds ratio = 8.13, 95% CI = 3.04 – 21.70

small study, therefore, failed to confirm the reported associations that were in the literature.

For the second example, let us suppose that we wish to examine the suggestion that diffuse idiopathic skeletal hyperostosis (DISH) is particularly common in people following the religious way of life, or are otherwise of 'high status'. The prevalence of DISH has been found to be higher among those buried at monastic sites than buried in lay cemeteries, and the reasons probably have to do with differences in the diet; DISH is associated nowadays with obesity and non-insulin-dependent diabetes, and this was probably also the case in the past.[15] Suppose that we have 43 cases of DISH, all males, and that we choose two controls at random from among the remaining males in the assemblages from which we have drawn the cases. We can then see how many might reasonably be said to be monks or other 'high-status' individuals, using criteria decided on at the start of the study. The findings are set out in Table 7.7. Here we can see that 18 of the cases were high status compared with only 7 of the controls, giving an M-H χ^2 of 20.7, an OR of 8.13 with a 95% CI of 3.04 – 21.70; all the results are highly significant and strongly suggest that the association is unlikely to have arisen by chance.[16]

Sample Sizes and Power of a Study

The object of analytical methods in epidemiology is to test an hypothesis; formally one is testing the null hypothesis (H_0), which states that there is *no* differences between cases and controls with respect to their exposure (or whatever measure is being examined). If, following appropriate statistical manipulation, the null hypothesis can be rejected, then it is reasonable to suppose that some explanation other than chance, and that is considered plausible (at least by the investigator), may explain the differences seen.[17] The unwary may commit one of two errors when testing the null hypothesis, as shown in Table 7.8. In the first case, a true null hypothesis is rejected,

Table 7.8   Type I and Type II errors

	True State of Null Hypothesis (H_0)	
Statistical Decision	H_0 true	H_0 false
Reject H_0	Type I error	Correct
Accept H_0	Correct	Type II error

giving rise to a false-positive result; this is referred to as a Type I error. In the second case, a false null hypothesis is accepted, thus providing a false-negative result; this – unsurprisingly – is known as a Type II error. The probability of a Type I error is designated by the Greek letter α; the probability of a Type II error is designated by the Greek β. The probability of a Type I error (α) is more familiar as the *significance level* (*p*), which is usually set at 0.05 (or 5%). A *p*-value of 5% indicates that there is only a 5% likelihood of having committed a Type I error and rejected a true null hypothesis. The probability of correctly rejecting a false null hypothesis (thus avoiding a Type II error) is known as the *power* of the study and is defined as $1 - \beta$. If the power of a study is low, there will be a good chance of committing a Type II error and coming up with inconclusive results. There is a trade-off in every type of study between protecting against Type I and Type II errors; the more you protect against Type I errors, the more likely you are to commit a Type II error.[18] This is the best way round, since getting a false-negative result generally has fewer consequences than getting a false-positive one.[19] It is possible to specify in advance the power of a study and the level of significance (most often set at 80% and 5%, respectively) and to use these numbers to calculate the sample sizes needed in a case-control study. In general, the larger the number of subjects, the greater the power of the study, but, at some point, the power of the study becomes saturated, and adding further numbers does not increase the power.[20]

Endnotes

1. For the most thorough account of this kind of study see: J. J. Schlesselman, *Case Control Studies: Design, Conduct, Analysis* (New York: Oxford University Press, 1982). It is rather more fashionable nowadays to use the term *case-referent*, rather than the older *case-control*, to reflect the fact that less emphasis is often placed on very tight matching. There is little harm in adhering to the original nomenclature, however.

2. M. J. Quinn, P. J. Babb, A. Brock, L. Kirby, and J. Jones, *Cancer Trends in England and Wales, 1950–1999* (London: The Stationary Office, 2001).

3. As we did, but even then with considerable difficulty. Those with solvent exposure were found to have a risk of contracting AML, which was 2–3 times that of the controls

[D. Lazarov, H. A. Waldron, and D. Pejin, 'Acute Myeloid Leukaemia and Exposure to Organic Solvents – A Case-Control Study', *European Journal of Epidemiology* 16 (2000): 295–301].

4. In modern case-control studies a bias may be introduced by using prevalent cases if the risk factor adversely affects survival, since the pool of prevalent cases will include few patients with a short survival time. This is sometimes known as Neyman's bias [G. Hill, J. Connolly, R. Herbert, J. Lindsay, and W. Millar, 'Neyman's Bias Revisited', *Journal of Clinical Epidemiology* 56 (2003): 292–96].

5. See, for example, Schlesselman, *Case Control Studies: Design, Conduct, Analysis* (New York: Oxford University Press, 1982), pp. 109–11; Rothman and Greenland, *Ibid.*, pp. 155–57. The short paper by J. M. Bland and D. G. Altman ['Matching', *British Medical Journal* 309 (1994): 1128] is also worth a read.

6. G. Liu, W. Zhou, and D. C. Christiani, 'Molecular Epidemiology of Non-Small Cell Lung Cancer', *Seminars in Respiratory and Critical Care Medicine* 26 (2005): 265–72.

7. C. L. Daly, 'Molecular Epidemiology: A Tool for Understanding Control of Tuberculosis Transmissions', *Clinics in Chest Medicine* 26 (2005): 217–31.

8. P. Hrelia, F. Maffei, S. Angelini, and G. C. Forti, 'A Molecular Epidemiological Approach to Health Risk Assessment of Urban Air Pollution', *Toxicology Letters* 149 (2004): 261–67; P. A. Schulte, 'Some Implications of Genetic Biomarkers in Occupational Epidemiology and Practice', *Scandinavian Journal of Work, Environment and Health* 30 (2004): 71–9.

9. The difficulties in proceeding from association to causation, and Bradford Hill's part in it, have already been discussed in Chapter 1.

10. See Schlesselman, *Case Control Studies: Design, Conduct, Analysis* (New York: Oxford University Press, 1982), pp. 58–63.

11. This is not the place to go into the technicalities of this or other procedures to deal with confounding. Those who wish to learn more about it should consult the original paper of N. Mantel and W. Haenszel, 'Statistical Aspects of the Analysis of Data from Retrospective Studies of Disease', *Journal of the National Cancer Institute* 22 (1959): 719–48; or Schlesselman, *Case Control Studies: Design, Conduct, Analysis* (New York: Oxford University Press, 1982), pp. 183–90; 254–63; and 275–80. The Mantel-Haenszel paper is the most often cited paper in the entire epidemiological literature.

12. A program for calculating the M-H chi-squared statistic is freely available from the website of the Centers for Disease Control and Prevention (CDC); Epi Info can be downloaded from www.cdc.gov.

13. See also, J. M. Bland and D. G. Altman, 'The Odds Ratio', *British Medical Journal* 320 (2000): 1468.

14. The references to these papers, and others mentioned in this section, can be found in my paper, 'A Case-Referent Study of Spondylolysis and Spina Bifida and Transitional Vertebrae in Human Skeletal Remains', *International Journal of Osteoarchaeology* 3 (1993): 55–7.

15. For further details see J. Rogers and T. Waldron, 'DISH and the Monastic Way of Life', *International Journal of Osteoarchaeology* 11 (2001): 357–65.

16. Epi Info will also calculate odds ratios and confidence intervals, in addition to the M-H chi-squared; if you have not done so already, download it now.

17. Authors are wonderfully creative at devising plausible explanations for associations that may at first sight seem unlikely and that may, in many cases, be due to confounding. This has been discussed in two interesting papers: G. D. Smith and A. N. Phillips, 'Confounding in Epidemiological Studies: Why "Independent" Effects May Not Be All That They Seem', *British Medical Journal* 305 (1992): 757–59 and G. D. Smith, A. N. Phillips, and J. D. Neaton, 'Smoking as an "Independent" Risk Factor for Suicide: Illustration of an Artifact from Observational Epidemiology?' *Lancet* 340 (1992): 709–12.

18. There is also a Type III error – sometimes also confusingly known as a Type 0 error – which, according to Howard Raiffa occurs when you get the right answer to the wrong question [*Decision Analysis* (Reading, MA: Addison-Wesley, 1968), p. 264]. See also S. Schwartz and K. M. Carpenter, 'The Right Answer for the Wrong Question: Consequences of Type III Error for Public Health Research', *American Journal of Public Health* 89 (1999): 1175–80. The Type IV error is defined as the incorrect interpretation of a correctly rejected null hypothesis [K. J. Ottenbacher, 'Statistical Conclusion Validity and Type IV Errors in Rehabilitation Research', *Archives of Physical and Medical Rehabilitation* 73 (1992): 121–25]. Finally, there is one other error – and one with which statisticians are only too familiar – that occurs when the test the statistician applies to collected data does not provide the answer the investigator wants and when the investigator then suggests an inappropriate analysis that he or she thinks *will* give the required answer. This is sometimes called a Type IX error.

19. One does need sometimes to be careful when interpreting 'negative' studies and remember that absence of evidence is not necessarily evidence of absence [D. G. Altman and J. M. 'Bland Have Words to Say about This: Absence of Evidence Is Not Evidence of Absence', *British Medical Journal* 311 (1995): 485]. The reader will not fail to have noticed the number of occasions on which reference is given to these two authors. They have compiled an invaluable series of short and easily understood *Statistics Notes*, which were originally all published in the *BMJ*. They are rather more conveniently also posted on the BMJ website: www.bmj.com.

20. The methods used to determine power and sample size can be found in, for example, J. L. Kelsey, A. S. Whittemore, A. S. Evans, and W. D. Thompson, *Methods in Observational Epidemiology*, 2nd ed. (New York: Oxford University Press, 1996) and P. Armitage, G. Berry, and J. N. S. Matthews, *Statistical Methods in Medical Research*, 4th ed. (Oxford: Blackwell, 2002). There are also several power calculators posted on the web or as part of statistical soft-ware packages. A useful nomogram for calculating power can be found in F. Whitley and J. Ball, 'Statistical Review 4: Sample Size Calculations', *Critical Care* 6 (2002): 335–41.

8 | A Question of Occupation

The August 1994 edition of the *Scientific American* shows a female skeleton from the Neolithic site of Abu Hureyra in Syria grinding grain on a saddle quern; the individual who actually undertook this task apparently was identified on the basis of common arthritic conditions affecting her skeleton, including the spine, knee, and the first metatarso-phalangeal joint.[1] An orthopaedic surgeon commenting in a later edition of the magazine said that the suggestion that these deformities resulted from grinding grain made 'little sense'.[2] Nor should this kind of *post hoc ergo propter hoc* reasoning make much sense to *anyone* who stops to think for a moment about it.

It is understandable that those who examine human remains should wish to deduce as much as possible about the lives of individuals from their skeletons, but this has led to some very extravagant claims being made about the role of environmental stresses, parity, social status, and occupation or occupationally related activities. In the case of occupation the claim to be able to reconstruct the type of work undertaken by a particular individual is frequently made in respect of the presence of osteoarthritic or other so-called degenerative diseases. Faced with a skeleton with diseased joints, some authors apparently cannot resist the urge to deduce an underlying unifying cause, and they frequently come up with the notion that the reason has to do with the individual's occupation. From this starting point, they then tell their readers what that occupation was with a confidence that borders on the startling. The extreme opposite of this interpretive view of palaeopathology lies with what one might call the nihilists, who consider that there is virtually nothing that can be gained from the examination of the skeleton, not always excluding age and sex. It may be dull to suggest that the truth probably lies somewhere between these two extremes, but there is no reason to suppose that the truth, when we know what it is, will always be interesting.

Were it really possible to be able to determine the occupation of past populations from the diseases that affect their skeletons, this would be immensely useful and would be of great value to the palaeoepidemiologist. And because the prospect is so alluring, the premises that underpin this assumption are not always carefully examined, or, if they are, the proponents of the idea have not always wished to advertise the conclusions very widely.

Since osteoarthritis is the condition that is most frequently interpreted in the light of possible occupational or activity-related factors, I propose to consider now whether there is any basis for supposing that occupation could, even under the most ideal circumstances, be derived from the pattern of osteoarthritis? Osteoarthritis is nowadays considered to be the end result of a number of different processes that interact to produce what is referred to as joint failure[3] manifested by the morphological appearances that are very well recognised as concomitants of this failure. Factors known to be important include a genetic predisposition, sex, age, race, obesity, trauma, and movement,[4] while more recent research suggests that there may also be a vascular component.[5] Movement is particularly important, because the supposition that underlies the presumed relationship between work and osteoarthritis is that the changes occur in those joints that are most used or perhaps subject to repeated trauma as the result of forceful movement. There is no denying that movement is a crucial factor in the development of the changes in osteoarthritis; joints that do not move, for whatever reason, do not get the disease, and so the idea apparently has some clinical validity.

In all instances in which relationships are being inferred between, say, nutritional status and skeletal changes, or life style and skeletal changes, a reasonable starting point seems to be always to defer to what is known from modern clinical or epidemiological studies. In the case of occupational arthropathy there is a copious literature, and a number of relationships have been proposed, many based on case studies and cross-sectional studies. There is also an extremely voluminous literature on the relationship between what is often referred to as 'rheumatism' and occupation and on musculoskeletal pain and occupation. It is important clearly to differentiate among osteoarthritis, rheumatism, and musculoskeletal pain in these studies. Unless otherwise specified, rheumatism in this context may be taken to mean soft tissue disease and not joint disease;[6] musculoskeletal pain may be the result of both soft tissue and joint disease, but there is generally no means of knowing which is the major cause, and so associations found between occupations and musculoskeletal pain should not be taken as suggestive of a relationship with osteoarthritis. The results of studies that refer either to rheumatism or musculoskeletal pain are evidently of no help to those studying disease in the skeleton, since neither can be diagnosed. The only modern studies that are of help to palaeoepidemiologists are those that concentrate specifically on osteoarthritis. In epidemiological as opposed to clinical studies, the presence of osteoarthritis depends on the radiological demonstration of features such as joint space narrowing and the presence of marginal osteophytes following the example of Lawrence in his now classic studies in the 1960s and 70s.[7]

Many occupations have been found to have an excess prevalence of osteoarthritis at some joint or other compared with a control group, and a few of these associations are shown in Table 8.1.[8] When examining the results of studies on occupational arthropathy, the investigator should bear some points in mind. Firstly, there is very little consistency about the results; for example, some authors find that coal miners have an increased prevalence of osteoarthritis of the spine, whereas others do not; that there are many negative studies in which *no* association is found between work and osteoarthritis;[9] that many people who work in strenuous occupations do not get osteoarthritis, and that many who work in sedentary occupations with little stress on their joints do develop the disease. Probably still the best demonstration of the relationship between work and osteoarthritis is that published by Hadler and his colleagues, who studied the pattern of osteoarthritis in the hands in women working in a worsted mill in Virginia. The women in the mill were engaged

Table 8.1   Some reported associations between osteoarthritis and occupation

Site(s) of Osteoarthritis	Occupation
Foot, knee	Ballet dancers
Wrist, elbow	Chipping and grinding operatives; Foundry workers
Metacarpo-phalangeal joints	Jackhammer operators
Knee	Labourers
Spine, knee	Miners
Hand	Mill workers
Hip	Farmers

principally in three tasks: spinning, burling, and winding. In all three groups of workers the dominant hand was more often affected than the nondominant hand, but the winders were much less likely to have osteoarthritis in the second and third digits than were burlers or spinners, and the spinners alone had no involvement of the fifth digit.[10]

Much more recently a relationship has become established between farming and the development of osteoarthritis of the hip. The association was first recognised in the 1990s[11] and has been confirmed in many studies since then. It has been established that farmers – whatever their principal activity – have a relative risk of developing osteoarthritis of the hip of about 9 compared with the general population.[12]

The overwhelming impression that one gets from reading the modern epidemiological literature is that very little convincing evidence indicates a *consistent* relationship between a particular occupation and a particular form of osteoarthritis; given the multifactorial nature of the condition, this is probably what one ought to expect. Perhaps the most that can be said is that some occupations in which repetitive and strenuous movements of some joints occur will determine which joints are affected in those genetically predisposed to the disease.

To judge from modern epidemiological work, then, I suggest that there is very little reason to suppose that occupation is related to osteoarthritis in any consistent or coherent manner, but let us accept that it is; under those circumstances could we infer an occupation from the pattern of osteoarthritis in the skeleton? In other words, can we argue from the outcome variable that is seen in the bone back to the proximate cause?

We might best start by considering some of the possibilities about the cause(s) of osteoarthritis. There seem to be to be four, which we could call the simple, plural, complex, and interactive models. The simple model (Figure 8.1a) states that there is one and only one cause of the disease; the plural model (Figure 8.1b) states that there are many causes, but they act independently of one another; the complex model also states that there are many causes, but that for the disease to be present, all must act together (Figure 8.1c); the interactive model states that there are different factors, but they interact in any combination to produce the outcome.

In the simple model (8a) there is only a single cause; in the multiple model (8b) there are several potential causes acting singly; in the complex model (8c) there are several causes that must all act together; and

(a)

(b)

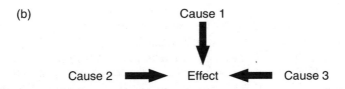

(c)

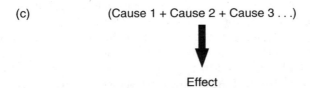

(d)

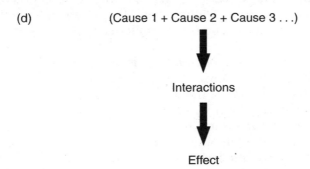

Figure 8.1 Various models of osteoarthritis

in the interactive model (8d) there are several causes any number of which interact to produce the disease.

What is abundantly clear from a consideration of these models is that palaeoepidemiologists, starting with the outcome and trying to reason backward to cause, could succeed *only* if the simple model were the correct one. That is to say, the cause of osteoarthritis could be inferred only if it were known that it had only a single cause. With the plural model, it would be impossible to say with any confidence which of the many causes was operating, and in the complex model, no inference could be made about which of the many causes, which have to act in concert, was having the dominant effect, if indeed it could be said that *any* was dominant.

We know, in fact, that osteoarthritis is a multifactorial disease, and so it is the interactive model that is most plausible. To try to determine which of the many factors is mainly responsible for the development of the disease is rather like looking at a bucket of water that was filled from several taps either singly or in combination and trying to say which way it really was done (Figure 8.2). It is pretty obvious that there is not the remotest chance of saying where the water in the bucket came from unless each tap delivers a different colour water, and even then the water will almost certainly be a mixture of colours. It is very unfortunate for palaeoepidemiologists that they are at the bucket end of the business when they need to be at the tap end – as their modern counterparts are – so that they can tell which of the taps is actually turned on.

The taps represent the various factors that interact to cause osteoarthritis; they are shown filling a bucket that represents the disease. It is impossible to tell which tap(s) filled the bucket merely by looking at the water in it. Methodologically, palaeoepidemiologists are at the bucket end, whereas their modern counterparts are at the tap end.

Since we know that occupation is *not* the sole cause of osteoarthritis, there is no chance of being able to deduce the former from the latter – no hope of tracing the water in the bucket back to one tap. If this were not discouragement enough, there is yet another matter that works against being able to do so. Even in those cases in which an occupationally related activity seems to be important in determining the expression of osteoarthritis, there are no unique features about the expression. Thus, osteoarthritis of the hands is not exclusive to worsted mill works, nor osteoarthritis of the hip to farmers; the majority of those who develop osteoarthritis at these sites will not be in these occupations, perhaps in no occupation at

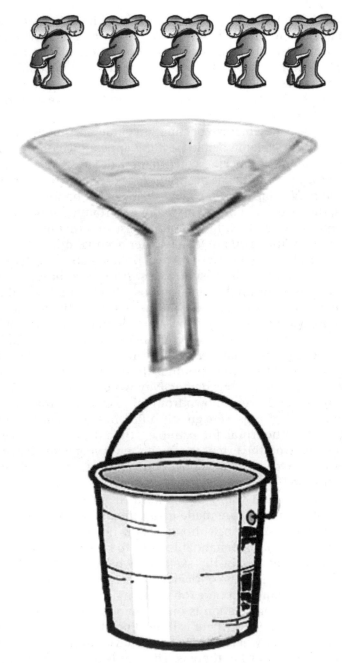

Figure 8.2 Taps and bucket model of osteoarthritis

all. Given a skeleton with osteoarthritis of the hip, and given that we believe farmers to have a relative risk of 9 for this disease, this still leaves us unable to say whether the skeleton before us was one of the hundreds of nonfarmers who might have had it.[13] We could guess the skeleton was that of a farmer and perhaps be correct, although there is no way of validating this assumption, and if we were right it would be for the wrong reasons.[14]

The only way in which an occupation could accurately be determined from the skeleton would be if the appearance of the disease at a single site, or a specific combination of sites, was unique to those following a particular occupation. If osteoarthritis of the hip presented *only* in farmers, or osteoarthritis of the hands *only* in mill workers, then we could be secure in our ascertainment of the occupation, but we know that this is not the case and that most of those with these conditions do not follow either occupation.[15]

There is a somewhat better prospect of being able to infer something about activity in assemblages from the basis of their osteoarthritis. For example, let us suppose that in one group there is a predominance of osteoarthritis of the hand, shoulder, and knee, whereas in another, separated by a considerable interval of time from the first, the major sites affected are the sterno-clavicular joint, the hip, and the foot; then clearly different factors are likely to have been operating in the two to produce these distinct patterns of disease. Of the factors to consider, activity would be one of the most significant, and if it were known from other evidence that the ways of life of the two groups were greatly different – one being an urban group and the other rural, for example – then it would be permissible to speculate on the extent to which the varying activities undertaken by the two groups might have contributed to the development of their disease.[16]

This brief account will, I hope, act to deter some of the more extravagant claims that are made about the ability to deduce occupation from the skeleton, although I am not overly optimistic.[17] There is a perfectly understandable drive to make the most of what little evidence survives in the skeleton, which sometimes has the effect of overwhelming the critical faculties. It would be possible to point to other examples where too much may be being made of too little, or where interpretation is outstripping hard evidence, and it generally happens where there is little clinical evidence to back up the suppositions or where the observers have not troubled to make themselves aware of what there is. The words of Thomas McKeown are apposite in this regard; he wrote:

In general... I am doubtful about the reliability of much historical evidence related to health, unless it has been screened critically through present-day experience.[18]

The same is true of palaeoepidemiological and palaeopathological evidence, and those who work in these fields ignore McKeown's stricture at their peril.

Endnotes

1. T. Molleson, The eloquent bones of Abu Hureya, *Scientific American*, August (1994): 60–5.

2. D. B. Mann, 'Picking at Bones', *Scientific American*, January (1995): 5.

3. G. Nuki, 'Ostoearthritis: A Problem of Joint Failure', *Zeitschrift für Rheumatologie* 58 (1999): 142–47.

4. P. Sarzi-Puttini, M. A. Cimmino, R. Scarpa, R. Caporali, F. Parazzine, A. Zaninelli, F. Atzenie, and B. Canesi, 'Osteoarthritis: An Overview of the Disease and Its Treatment Strategies', *Seminars in Arthritis and Rheumatism* 35 (2005): (Supplement 1), 1–10.

5. P. G. Conaghan, H. Vanharanta, and P. A. Dieppe, 'Is Progressive Osteoarthritis an Atheromatous Vascular Disease?' *Annals of the Rheumatic Diseases* 64 (2005): 1539–41.

6. Although now rather old, J. A. D. Anderson's review of soft-tissue rheumatism and occupation remains the most comprehensive and best: 'Rheumatism in Industry: A Review', *British Journal of Industrial Medicine* 28 (1990): 103–21.

7. Lawrence published many studies on the epidemiology of osteoarthritis and the relationship with occupation. His main results are summarised in J. S. Lawrence, *Rheumatism in Populations* (London: Heinemann Medical Books, 1977). This book contains references to the original papers and is an excellent source for those who wish to consult them. Lawrence and his colleagues undertook a number of cross-sectional studies of general population samples, taking X rays of many joints in the same individuals. It is almost certain that studies such as his, which required considerable X-ray exposure to normal subject, would not be permitted nowadays with our much stricter control of exposure to radiation. On this account there is little prospect that Lawrence's studies will be repeated or extended. When attempting to apply results, especially any prevalence data, to past populations, remember that different criteria were used to diagnose osteoarthritis than are likely to be used to diagnose the disease in the skeleton.

8. Kennedy produced a much larger table of modern epidemiological studies up to the late 1980s. It can be found in K. A. R. Kennedy, 'Skeletal Markers of Occupational Stress', in *Reconstruction of Life from the Skeleton*, M. Y. Işcan and K. A. R. Kennedy, eds. (New York: Alan Liss, 1989), pp. 129–60. The table occupies no less than 15 pages of the chapter, but since little is said about the quality of the studies included there, the reader will need to refer back to the original papers to derive much benefit from it; it does, however, save the interested reader a great deal of time searching through old databases.

9. It is generally more difficult to have a paper with negative results published than one with positive results, and this fact leads to a certain amount of publication bias: in any

discipline are always more papers with positive than with negative findings. This bias assumes some importance when reviews are undertaken and where the strength of an association may be deduced by balancing the number of positive and negative results (usually deduced from the value of the odds ratios reported); in any such process the positives are likely to outweigh the negatives. To try to overcome this type of bias, many statistical reviews – so-called meta-analyses – try to be as careful as possible to include negative as well as positive studies, often appealing to authors of unpublished papers to make their negative results available to them.

10. Hadler's observations are contained in two excellent papers and are further summarised in a book chapter; all are worth consulting. See N. M. Hadler, 'Industrial Rheumatology: Clinical Investigations into the Influence of the Pattern of Usage on the Pattern of Regional Musculoskeletal Disease, *Arthritis and Rheumatism* 20 (1977): 1019–25; N. M. Hadler, D. B. Gillings, H. R. Imbus, P. M. Levitin, D. Makuc, P. D. Utsinger, W. J. Yount, D. Slusser, and N. Moskovitz, 'Hand Structure and Function in an Industrial Setting: Influence of Three Patterns of Stereotyped Repetitive Usage, *Arthritis and Rheumatism* 21 (1978): 210–20; N. M. Hadler, 'The Variable of Usage in the Epidemiology of Osteoarthritis', in *Epidemiology of Osteoarthritis*, J. G. Peyron, ed. (London: Geigy, 1980), pp. 164–71.

11. C. Cooper, 'Occupational Activity and the Risk of Osteoarthritis', *Journal of Rheumatology* 43 (1995): Supplement 10–12.

12. Among the many papers on this subject, those that best summarise the results are probably A. Lievense, S. Bierma-Zeinstra, A. Verhagen, J. Verhaar, and B. Koes, 'Influence of Work on the Development of Osteoarthritis of the Hip: A Systematic Review', *Journal of Rheumatology* 28 (2001): 2520–28; K. Walker-Bone and K. T. Palmer, 'Musculoskeletal Disorders in Farmers and Farm Workers', *Occupational Medicine (London)* 52 (2002): 441–50; J. S. Schouten, R. A. de Bie, and G. Swaen, 'An Update on the Relationship between Occupational Factors and Osteoarthritis of the Hip and Knee, *Current Opinion in Rheumatology* 14 (2002): 89–92. The relationship was considered to be so well established that in 2002 the Industrial Injuries Advisory Council in the United Kingdom recommended making osteoarthritis of the hip in farmers a prescribed industrial disease, in other words, one that attracted a small amount of compensation from the government. [For the Council's deliberations see: Department of Work and Pensions, *Osteoarthritis of the Hip, Command 597* (London: HMSO, 2002)]. It is interesting that the reason that farmers seem more at risk of osteoarthritis of the hip has *not* been established, although there is a general inclination to blame heavy lifting as the cause. This does not seem entirely plausible given that most heavy jobs on the farm are now mechanised and that farmers are at seemingly at risk irrespective of whether they are agricultural, dairy, or mixed farmers. Luckily for the modern epidemiologists, it seems clear that more work needs to be done to clarify the cause of this association.

13. In this context, the distinction needs to be made between relative and absolute risk. Thus, suppose that the prevalence of osteoarthritis of the hip among the general population is 1 per 1,000; then with a relative risk of 9, the prevalence among farmers would be 9 per 1,000. The *absolute* risk, however, is still small (*ca.* 1%), and the great majority of farmers would go through their lives without contracting the disease.

14. Unfortunately there is no way of knowing how likely a guess is to be correct. The chance that an individual skeleton belongs to a particular occupational group is n/N, where n = number of individuals in the occupational group and N = number in the

total work force. Neither the number nor the likelihood of guessing correctly can be known, but we can be sure that the chances are vanishingly small.

15. For those who still believe that they might be able to determine the occupation of an individual from the skeleton let me ask them to imagine that they are in the rheumatology clinic of a general hospital and that they have access only to the X rays of the patients who have osteoarthritis at the clinic that day. They are assured that the X rays show all the joints affected by the disease, and their task is to say what the occupation of each patient is. I doubt that many would be prepared to put much money on their answers being correct, yet this is, in effect, what they are trying to do with the skeleton.

16. Whether osteoarthritis is the best marker to use for deducing patterns of activity in an assemblage is by no means certain, but this is not the place to enter into that discussion. Suffice it to say that the pattern of enthesophytes may be more sensitive – in the absence of some other diseases. These occur at tendon insertions that may have been subjected to trauma consequent on continual forced repetitive movements. The pattern of enthesophytes within an assemblage may provide better evidence of activity than osteoarthritis, but to date little work has been undertaken; see, for example O. Dutour, 'Enthesopathies (Lesions of Muscular Insertions) as Indicators of the Activities of Neolithic Saharan populations', *American Journal of Physical Anthropology* 71 (1986): 221–24; E. Brubezy, J. Goulet, J. Bruzek, J. Jelinek, D. Rouge, and B. Ludes, 'Epidemiology of Osteoarthritis and Enthesopathies in a European Population Dating Back 7700 Years, *Joint, Bone, Spine* 69 (2002): 580–88.

17. Those who favour the interpretive method of palaeopathology are fond of referring to Sherlock Holmes, especially his remarks to the hapless Lestrade in *A Study in Scarlet*, when he helpfully advised Lestrade that the murderer in the case 'was a man. He was more than six feet high, was in the prime of life, had small feet for his height, wore coarse, square-toed boots and smoked a Trinchinopoly cigar.... In all probability the murderer had a florid face, and the fingernails of his right hand were remarkably long'. What they tend to forget is that Conan Doyle (and hence, Holmes himself) knew the answers in advance, and we are not told of the many occasions when Holmes must have got it wrong had he been a mere mortal.

18. T. McKeown, *The Origins of Human Disease* (Oxford: Blackwell, 1988), p. 10.

9 | Planning a Study

Whatever the matter being investigated, it is likely that any palaeoepidemiological study is a variant on one of the three types described in earlier chapters; a cross-sectional study; a ranking study; or a case-control study. Irrespective of the type of study, the study must be well planned, well conducted, and well analysed so that the results are valid and thus provide information that is helpful in understanding disease in the past. In this final chapter I identify some important features of any epidemiological study.

I do assume that the purpose of the study has been carefully considered and is clear in the minds of the investigators. If it is proposed to seek money to fund the study, prospective applicants should be aware that there are – regrettably – rather few sources to which application can be made and that invariably the prime requirement is that the application is presented in the form of an hypothesis to be tested; if the grant-giving body is one that supports archaeological rather than medical research – and this will almost certainly be the case – then the hypothesis has to be generated in the form of an archaeological rather than a medical question, and to fulfil this criterion may require a bit of creative formulation on the part of the applicants.[1]

The Study-Base

Let us further assume that the hypothesis has been formulated and that there is no financial barrier to carrying out the study; then the first task is to identify the study-base, and it is here that palaeoepidemiologists suffer most by comparison with their colleagues who carry out studies on the living (or recently dead). In effect, the study-base is largely chosen for you. For example, if you wish to test whether fractures of the ankle are more common in rural rather than urban assemblages, then the study-base can be selected only from assemblages that are already above ground and that are sufficiently large to provide the numbers required, whatever they may be. This scarcity of suitable material accounts for the frequent appearance of some assemblages in the literature.[2] Unfortunately there seems to be no way round this since to excavate an assemblage *de novo* would almost certainly prove to be not only too expensive an undertaking and too time consuming, but there also would be no guarantee of the quality or the quantity of the material recovered. We should perhaps not dwell on the nonrandom nature of the assemblages; otherwise, the temptation will be to devote ourselves to other matters entirely. We must be satisfied that there are *any* assemblages at all to study, given that it is only relatively recently that human remains have been carefully and properly recovered, preserved, and curated and given the attention they deserve.

The first step toward establishing the study-base is to decide on the inclusion criteria for entry into the study. These criteria *must* be determined at the planning stage, preferably written down, and strictly adhered to as the study progresses so as to avoid selection bias. In a prevalence study, carefully consider the denominator; it will be different for studying the prevalence of osteoarthritis of the hip or the prevalence of spondylolysis, for example. For the first example, the inclusion criteria require that only adult skeletons with hip joints are admitted (or a single diseased hip joint if only one is present), whereas for the second, only skeletons with the lumbar spine present would be admissible.[3]

For a case-control study, the criteria by which a case will be ascertained need to be determined in advance; this may not be as easy as it sounds, since it depends on detecting the presence of some outcome variable that will itself have to be defined, as described later. The controls will, of course, be selected from among the remainder of the assemblage who do not fit the criteria for being a case. Almost certainly some form of matching will be required, but think carefully to make sure that matching really is necessary, since any form of matching inevitably reduces the pool of available controls. Matching on age and sex is obviously required when studying a condition that is age and/or sex dependent, but when this is not the case, matching on these criteria may not be necessary. It is, therefore, essential to understand the nature of the condition or disease to be studied in order that matching not be done unnecessarily. The method for drawing controls should ensure – so far as is practicable – that each skeleton with the potential for inclusion in the study has an equal chance of being selected. This may be done, for example, with the use of random number tables from which a list of skeleton numbers can be drawn up; each of the skeletons selected is then examined to see whether other matching criteria are satisfied, and this procedure continues until the requisite number of controls is obtained. A simpler method and one that certainly is less time consuming would be to generate a list of all the skeletons in the assemblage that are not cases in the order of their given number and work through this list until all the controls have been obtained. The rationale for this approach is that there is likely to be no bias in the way in which the skeleton numbers have been allocated.[4] The number of controls required to give the study the appropriate power to determine that an odds ratio is significantly different from unity should be calculated in advance[5] using one of the formulae available for the purpose.[6] If, in order to avoid a Type II error, the number of controls required exceeds the number potentially available, move on to study another problem.[7]

In ranking studies, there are no problems either with denominator data or controls, but the issue of outcome variables is as crucial as it is to any other kind of study, and it is to these that we must now turn.

Outcome Variables

The prime object of any study is an outcome variable of some sort, frequently a disease or condition such as tuberculosis, spondylolysis, or Paget's disease. Whatever the outcome, however, the method of diagnosing or recognising it must be considered when the study is being planned, and the means by which this will be done must be agreed on, written down, and adhered to closely throughout the study so as to minimise selection bias. The most appropriate way to do this is to create an operational definition that, in the case of a pathological condition, should be based on what is known about it from the clinical literature. There is no point in basing the diagnosis of, let us say, iron deficiency anaemia on the basis of changes in the skull that are not recognised clinically, or of scurvy in juveniles on changes that are not accompanied by the pathognomonic radiological features in the long bones. Regrettably there are few conditions that afflict the skeleton that have pathognomonic signs, but where there are – eburnation in osteoarthritis or the radiological 'flame sign' in Paget's disease, for example – clearly these should have their place in the operational definition. Otherwise, a list of signs will have to be established using all the available evidence (and that may not be very much) and these (and only these) used to diagnose the condition in the skeleton. For the diagnosis of a sero-negative erosive arthropathy to be made, for example, it would be necessary that the following signs be present: erosions around or within a joint; changes in the sacroiliac joints (inflammatory signs or fusion); and spinal fusion. The requirement for all three signs to be present means that incomplete skeletons would probably not be available for inclusion in the study, and it is likely that the number of cases in any epidemiological study of human remains would be an underestimate of the true prevalence.

It is not at all easy always to come up with a satisfactory operational definition, and, even having done so, it may not be easy to adhere to it, especially if the number of cases in the study-base appears to be disappointingly small as the study proceeds. The temptation then is to relax the criteria so that more cases can be included. Under some circumstances this may be a reasonable approach, and there are instances in which it may be sensible to revise the criteria if they seem to be unrealistically stringent. If this *is* done, however, the study will have to be started again and all the material reexamined in the light of the revised criteria.

Rating Scales

Rating scales are often used to categorise changes in the skeleton, whether they be pathological changes or normal variants, but before choosing to use one in a study, consider what additional information its use will provide to the study. Is anything to be gained by grading the size of marginal osteophytes around a joint, or the degree of calculus on the teeth, or the size of Schmorl's nodes? If there *is* some clinical validity for grading changes, then that, of course, is reason enough to do so, but the number of occasions on which this will be the case are likely to very few indeed. Do not suppose that grading will somehow improve the quality of the data, since others will not likely be able to replicate the grading system without reference material or some objective means by which to do so. For scoring dental nonmetric traits, for example, casts are available for use with the Arizona State University Dental Anthropological System,[8] but there are no standards by which to judge pathological changes in the skeleton, so far as I am aware.[9] My advice is never to use a rating scale unless there seems to be no way of avoiding doing so, and, even then, register your objection in advance.

Data Collection

Collecting data will almost certainly occupy the most time in an epidemiological study, sometimes even surpassing the amount of time spent applying for and waiting for the award of a grant. When the study starts, avoid observer bias by adhering to protocols and procedures agreed to at the start of the study, and, when possible, use check lists to ensure compliance with selection criteria and operational definitions. Before proceeding with the main study, you might want to undertake a pilot study to test the inter- or intraobserver error rates. Do not be fooled, either, into thinking that the use of a single observer adds strength to the study; it usually has the opposite effect. For example, a study to test the validity of published methods for diagnosing a particular condition may indicate that the method is fallible; if only a single observer undertook the study, however, it will be impossible to counter the obvious criticism that it is not the method but the observer who is at fault. But if several observers come to the same conclusion, it seems more likely than not that the method truly should be consigned to oblivion, or at least revised to make it more useful.

Interobserver and intraobserver errors should be assessed on material that will not form part of the main study, and the error rates can be analysed using the kappa (κ) statistic referred to in Chapter 3. There are no absolute values for determining when agreement between observers is satisfactory, but most authors tend to defer to the scheme proposed by Landis and Koch[10] (see Table 9.1) or to the recommendations of Fleiss.[11] Generally one should aim for a value of κ of at least 0.80, but if the results of the test are not satisfactory, then the reasons for this should be examined, further training given as necessary, and the test repeated until the level of agreement is within the acceptable range.

Table 9.1 Levels of agreement indicated by various values of kappa (after Landis and Koch 1977)

Value of Kappa	Level of Agreement
≤ 0	Poor
0 – 0.20	Slight
0.21 – 0.40	Fair
0.41 – 0.60	Moderate
0.61 – 0.80	Substantial
0.81 – 1.00	Almost perfect

It should be obvious that any testing of intra- or interobserver error should be carried out *before* the main study is begun, but personal experience shows that this is by no means always the case. Having gathered all their data, some observers hit on the brilliant idea that perhaps it would be useful to include a note on observer error in their paper – sometimes at the suggestion of a helpful referee. Consternation follows when the results of that exercise show that the error rate in the test is so great that it obviates any conclusions that might have been drawn, and a search is made for a journal whose referees will overlook this trivial point.[12]

Analysis

The ways in which the collected data are to be analysed should be decided *in advance.* In many studies the end result is a simple 2 x 2 table that is analysed using a chi-squared test or by calculating an odds ratio. Many epidemiologists who undertake studies on the living find it very hard to come to terms with the fact that most epidemiological studies do not require complicated statistics, and so they overanalyse the data to a considerable degree. They often do so because their initial analyses fail to provide the required value for p or a confidence interval that does not include unity and urge their statistician onward to the correct answer, thereby committing a Type IX error. It is generally the case that there is much virtue in simplicity and that if simple tests do not show significant (that is, in the biological sense) differences, there are not likely to be any.[13]

If those who are planning a study have any doubts about their statistical competence (and probably even if they do not), then it is sensible to consult a statistician to discuss the aims of the study, the data that are to be collected, and to take advice on the best form of analysis to use. It can also be a very gratifying experience, since the statistician is likely to be so amazed to have been asked for his or her opinion before the study is completed that you are bound to get undivided attention. Once it has been decided how the data are to be analysed, then there should properly be no deviation from the decided approach, even though the results may not be as one would like. What statisticians hate is to be presented with a set of data that have already gone through the mill and be asked to find a significant (in the statistical sense) result. Under these circumstances, the statistician should rightly refer you to the wise and often quoted words of the great R. A. Fisher: 'To consult the statistician after an experiment is finished is often merely to ask him to conduct a *post mortem* examination. He can perhaps say what the experiment died of'.[14] No amount of statistical manipulation will improve the quality of poor data, and much misery can be avoided by including a statistician in the team devising the study protocol.[15]

Comparing Data

When the results of a palaeoepidemiological study have been obtained, it is often of interest to compare them with the results of other studies of your own, with modern studies, or with studies carried out by other observers. Comparing the results of different studies carried out by the same observers should be straightforward, although it is important to make sure that the same protocols and procedures have been followed in each case so that the results really are comparable. Comparison with modern studies is much more problematic. Apart from dealing with the inherent difficulties that may arise from comparing results in the living and the dead, modern studies of disease use very different methods to select their study-base. For example, recent studies of the incidence and prevalence of osteoarthritis of the knee have used discharge data of patients receiving surgery,[16] a questionnaire sent to a random sample of those living in Oxfordshire[17] or to patients selected from general practitioners' lists,[18] a case-control study of patients on a single general practice list,[19] radiography of a sample selected randomly from a community in China,[20] siblings,[21] and men in different occupations.[22] Trying to chose which – if any – of these results might be appropriate for comparison with an archaeological assemblage is an almost impossible task, and, in general, one can safely assume that there will be few if any modern prevalence data that can reliably be compared with palaeoepidemiological data. And, of course, incidence data will seldom be compatible with those obtained from a study of human remains. Radiographic studies of a general population sample are probably the most useful, but even then the criteria used to diagnose disease are likely to be different from those in palaeopathology. Thus, in osteoarthritis the degree of joint space narrowing and the presence of marginal osteophyte are used for a radiographic diagnosis[23] that would almost certainly result in a higher prevalence being recorded than when the palaeoepidemiological operational definition (the presence of eburnation) is used.

In some case, however, modern data can be used to compare the qualitative features of some diseases, if not their quantitative ones. For example, the increase of Paget's disease in the elderly and the higher prevalence in males than in females[24] could be confirmed in a skeletal assemblage, and there are other instances in which similar features could be compared even though the prevalence data themselves were not quantitatively comparable.

On some occasions it may be desirable to compare data with those published by other workers, and in this case somewhat different constraints apply. First and foremost investigators must satisfy themselves that the data to be compared are truly compatible: that is, are the age classes and the diagnostic criteria the same in each; have prevalences been correctly calculated; and are the raw data given so that further calculations can be made? From what I know of the literature, it is more likely that the moon is made of green cheese than that all these requirements will be satisfied.[25] Rather than turning to another problem, it is sometimes worth writing to the authors of papers that you would like to include in your analyses to ask whether the data can be provided. A courteous approach does sometimes produce the most unexpected results, but the hit rate is not likely to be great, and many authors may not reply, fearing the worst if their data fall into the wrong hand. If you do propose to use another author's raw data, it is at least polite to suggest a joint publication; such a suggestion may not only show you to be a considerate colleague but actually facilitate the release of the data to you.

At the present time, the prospects of being able to carry out much comparative work on published data are slim, and one of the purposes of writing this book is to encourage a discussion on the best way to record, analyse, and report palaeoepidemiological data and – sublime thought – perhaps arrive at a consensus; like Pindar's soul, we should exhaust the realm of the possible.[26]

Endnotes

1. The grant application tends to be a highly imaginative creation, seldom followed in the prosecution of a study. Like the published papers that may follow from a successful grant – as Richard Feynman said – there is seldom any place to say what you actually did (or are going to do) to achieve your ends [R. Feynman, Nobel Lecture 11 December 1965, in *Nobel Lectures, Physics 1963–1970* (Amsterdam: Elsevier, 1972), pp. 155–77].

2. In studies from the United Kingdom, the assemblages from Wharram Percy, Barton-on-Humber, and Christ Church Spitalfields appear with great frequency as a search of online databases will quickly confirm, whereas studies of ageing and sexing methods seem to be impossible to conduct without reference to the ubiquitous Terry collection (and to a lesser extent, the Todd Collection).

3. In this example, it might not be necessary for all the lumbar vertebrae to be present in every case, since the prevalence could be calculated separately for each vertebra.

4. In some circumstances this method will *not* be appropriate. For example, skeletons will probably be numbered in the order in which they are excavated, and so those buried later (and recovered earlier in the excavation) tend to be given numbers earliest in the sequence. If the study is examining the possibility that the condition under study was more common in one period that in another, clearly this method of selecting controls *would* introduce a bias.

5. This is a crucial point: the power of the study should *never* be calculated after data collection is complete. If it is then found that the power of the study is not sufficient for the purpose, nothing can be done about it [S. N. Goodman and J. A. Berlin, 'The Use of Predicted Confidence Intervals When Planning Experiments and the Misuse of Power When Interpreting Results', *Annals of Internal Medicine* 121 (1994): 200–06].

6. See, for example, M. D. Edwards, 'Sample Size Requirement for Case-Control Study Designs', *BMC Medical Research Methodology* 1 (2001): 11 and the corrections published in *BMC Medical Research Methodology* 2 (2002): 16. (This is an electronic journal; the full text can be downloaded from www.biomedcentral.com.) Many published studies do lack the necessary power to detect relative differences of 25% or even 50% [D. Moher, C. S. Dulberg, and G. A. Wells, 'Statistical Power, Sample Size, and Their Reporting in Randomized Controlled Trials', *Journal of the American Medical Association* 272 (1994): 122–24].

7. It is worth bearing in mind, however, that it is rarely worth choosing more than three controls per case, but even three may be difficult to recruit from some assemblages [J. M. Taylor, 'Choosing the Number of Controls in a Matched Case-Control Study: Some Sample Size, Power and Efficiency Considerations', *Statistics in Medicine* 5 (1986): 29–36].

8. C. G. Turner, C. R. Nichol, and G. R. Scott, 'Scoring Procedures for Key Morphological Traits of the Permanent Dentition, in *Advances in Dental Anthropology*, M. A. Kelly and C. S. Larsen, eds. (New York: Wiley-Liss, 1991), pp. 13–31.

9. The use of these rating scales can generate a vast amount of data – up to 300 items per set of teeth, which makes analysis so complicated that even when the scales are used, the results are most often dichotomised into present or absent, which rather negates their use in the first place!

10. J. R. Landis and G. G. Koch, 'The Measurement of Observer Agreement for Categorical Data', *Biometrics* 33 (1977): 159–74.

11. Fleiss considers that a kappa value greater than 0.75 represents excellent agreement; anything less than 0.4, however, is poor [J. Fleiss, *Statistical Methods for Rates and Proportions*, 2nd ed. (New York: J. Wiley & Sons, 1981), p. 218].

12. There are no grounds for optimism when it comes to diagnosing common conditions found in the skeleton. For example, a study in which observers were asked to note pathological changes in a series of 10 specimens all chosen to have osteoarthritis found that in only half the cases was eburnation noted despite the fact that the presence of eburnation was the criterion by which all the specimens had been chosen. The observers rated their level of expertise in palaeopathology; those who rated themselves as experts were unanimous that osteoarthritis was present in only 3 of the 10 specimens, whereas beginners were unanimous only about a single specimen. [For further details see T. Waldron and J. Rogers, 'Inter-observer Variation in Coding Osteoarthritis in Human Skeletal Remains', *International Journal of Osteoarchaeology* 1 (1991): 49–56]. A later study showed an accuracy of only about 29% in diagnosing different conditions in the skeleton [E. Miller, B. D. Ragsdale, and D. J. Ortner,

'Accuracy of Dry Bone Diagnosis: A Comment on Palaeopathological Methods, *International Journal of Osteoarchaeology* 6 (1996): 221–29]. These results do nothing to lessen the absolute requirement for checking methodology before embarking on an epidemiological study of any kind.

13. A paper by an eminent medical statistician is worth consulting on this point even though it is not strictly germane to the study of the dead: S. J. Pocock, 'The Simplest Statistical Test: How to Check for a Difference between Treatments', *British Journal of Medicine* 332 (2006): 1256–58.

14. R. A. Fisher, 'Presidential Address to the First Indian Statistical Conference, Calcutta', *Sankhyā* 4 (1938): 14–17.

15. I might also add that there is no harm in consulting an epidemiologist early on also if the level of expertise within the group is recognised not to be of the requisite standard. When reading through the literature relating to studies on both ancient and modern material, it does not take one long to come to the conclusion that these suggestions are widely ignored.

16. C. Mehrotra, P. L. Rimington, T. S. Naimi, W. Washington, and R. Miller, 'Trends in Total Knee Replacement Surgeries and Implications for Public Health, 1990–2000', *Public Health Reports* 120 (2005): 278–82.

17. L. Linsell, J. Dawson, K. Zondervan, P. Rose, A. Carr, T. Randall, and R. Fitzpatrick, 'Population Survey Comparing Older Adults with Hip versus Knee Pain in Primary Care', *British Journal of General Practice* 55 (2005): 192–98.

18. F. Salaffi, R. De Angelis, and W. Grassi, 'Prevalence of Musculoskeletal Conditions in an Italian Population Sample: Results of a Regional Community-Based Study. I: The MAPPING Study', *Clinical and Experimental Rheumatology* 23 (2005): 819–28.

19. J. Bedson, K. Jordan, and P. Croft, 'The Prevalence and History of Knee Osteoarthritis in General Practice: A Case-Control Study', *Family Practice* 22 (2005): 103–08.

20. H. Du, S. L. Chen, C. D. Bao, X. D. Wang, Y. Lu, Y. Y. Gu, J. R. Xu, W. M. Chai, J. Chen, H. Nakamura, and K. Nishioka, 'Prevalence and Risk Factors for Knee Osteoarthritis in Juang-Pa District, Shanghai, China', *Rheumatology International* 25 (2005): 585–90.

21. R. L. Neame, K. Muir, S. Doherty, and M. Doherty, 'Genetic Risk of Knee Osteoarthritis: A Sibling Study', *Annals of the Rheumatic Diseases* 63 (2004): 1022–27.

22. B. Jarvholm, S. Lewold, H. Malchau, and E. Vingard, 'Age, Bodyweight, Smoking Habits and the Risk of Severe Osteoarthritis in the Hip and Knee in Men', *European Journal of Epidemiology* 20 (2005): 537–42.

23. An atlas of changes in the knee has been published to try to standardise the recording of osteoarthritis at this site [Y. Nagaosa, M. Mateus, B. Hassan, P. Lanyon, and M. Doherty, 'Development of a Logically Devised Line Drawing Atlas for Grading Knee Osteoarthritis', *Annals of the Rheumatic Diseases* 59 (20): 587–95].

24. J. P. Walsh, 'Paget's Disease of Bone', *Medical Journal of Australia* 181 (2004): 262–65.

25. It is not always the fault of the authors that raw data are not published; editors jealous of the space made available to them by their publishers seldom permit the publication of raw data in any quantity.

26. Pythian Odes, III, p. 109.

10 Last Words

The examination of human remains has given me – and gives to many others – a great deal of satisfaction, and that in itself is sufficient reason to pursue it. There is a greater source of satisfaction, however, in knowing that, to whatever small degree, one is adding to the knowledge of and understanding of our ancestors; we might also on some – admittedly rather rare occasions – be able to contribute to the understanding of the natural history of disease, and this may have relevance to those who study disease only in a modern context. If we intend our study to have the latter purpose, more stringent criteria are required in the interpretation and presentation of our observations, and one hopes that the ideas set out in this book will go some way toward achieving these ends.

Some readers may object that the emphasis throughout has been too restrictive, with too little allowance made for interpretation; they may perhaps say with Sydney Smith (the pathologist, not the cleric and wit; the pathologist was certainly not much of a wit) that 'My report was partly speculative... but without speculation it would not have been much use.'[1] And, of course, it is idle – even perverse – to suggest that one can advance any subject without interpretation and speculation. Writing about the role of the historian, Isaiah Berlin reminds us: 'That to exercise their proper function [they] require the capacity for imaginative insight, without which the bones of the past remain dry and lifeless. To deploy it is, and always has been, a risky business'.[2] It is the risks attached to imaginative insight that I am anxious to point out; interpretation and speculation are fine so long as their bounds are confined by the limits of the observations on which they are based and by our own experience and that of others, who are perhaps wiser than we are. Let me close with Isaiah Berlin again: in his essay on Vico, who was one of the most original thinkers of the eighteenth century, he writes: 'The crucial role he [Vico] assigns to the imagination must not blind us – and did not blind him – to the necessity for verification; he allows that critical methods of examining evidence are indispensable.'[3]

Critical methods for examining evidence are no less dispensable in palaeoepidemiology than in any other field of serious human endeavour.

Endnotes

1. S. Smith, *Mostly Murder* (London: Harrap, 1959), p. 15.

2. I. Berlin, 'Giambattista Vico and Cultural History', in *The Crooked Timber of Humanity* (London: Fontana Press, 1991), p. 69.

3. I. Berlin, *Ibid.*, p. 64.

Index

Note: Italicized page numbers refer to tables.

About the Author

Tony Waldron combines medicine with archaeology; he is a consultant physician at St Mary's Hospital in London and a visiting professor at the Institute of Archaeology, University College London. He previously taught epidemiology for several years at the London School of Hygiene and Tropical Medicine and carried out research on neurotoxicology. He was for several years editor of the *British Journal of Industrial Medicine*. In recent years he has examined the application of epidemiological techniques to the study of human remains, with special reference to the joint diseases. He enjoyed a very profitable collaboration with the late Juliet Rogers in Bristol and wrote a *Field Guide to Joint Disease in Archaeology* with her. In 1991 he cofounded the *International Journal of Osteoarchaeology* with Ann Stirland and coedited the journal for the first 10 years. His present research interests are in the epidemiology of infectious diseases and tumours in human remains, and in growth and development. He has published several books on medical and archaeological topics and over 250 research papers.